AF694816

PICTURING WOMEN'S HEALTH

Warwick Series in the Humanities

Series Editor: Tim Lockley

Titles in this Series

1 Classicism and Romanticism in Italian Literature: Leopardi's *Discourse on Romantic Poetry*
Fabio A. Camilletti

2 Rome, Postmodern Narratives of a Cityscape
Dom Holdaway and Filippo Trentin (eds)

3 Gender and Space in Rural Britain, 1840–1920
Gemma Goodman and Charlotte Mathieson (eds)

Forthcoming Titles

Knowing Nature in Early Modern Europe
David Beck (ed.)

PICTURING WOMEN'S HEALTH

EDITED BY

Francesca Scott, Kate Scarth and Ji Won Chung

Routledge
Taylor & Francis Group
LONDON AND NEW YORK

First published 2014 by Pickering & Chatto (Publishers) Limited

2 Park Square, Milton Park, Abingdon, Oxfordshire OX14 4RN
52 Vanderbilt Avenue, New York, NY 10017

Routledge is an imprint of the Taylor & Francis Group, an informa business

First issued in paperback 2019

BRITISH LIBRARY CATALOGUING IN PUBLICATION DATA

Picturing women's health. – (Warwick series in the humanities)
1. Women – Health and hygiene – History – 19th century. 2. Women – Health and hygiene – History – 19th century – Sources.
I. Series II. Scarth, Kate, editor. III. Scott, Francesca, editor. IV. Chung, Ji Won, editor.
613'.04244'09034-dc23

ISBN-13: 978-1-8489-3424-5 (hbk)
ISBN-13: 978-0-367-87595-4 (pbk)

Typeset by Pickering & Chatto (Publishers) Limited

CONTENTS

ACKNOWLEDGEMENTS

Picturing Women's Health sprang from a shared research interest that spanned three very different theses at the University of Warwick. The three editors, who have since gone their separate ways, have been bound by this project for several years, and now feel some sadness (if not also a little relief) as it draws to a close. They have been guided, first and foremost, by Jacqueline Labbe, a remarkable scholar who continues to offer kindness, encouragement and thoughtful advice to each individually, and to whom they feel they owe the most.

The conference that inspired this collection was kindly supported by the British Association for Romantic Studies, the History of Medicine and the Humanities Research Centre at Warwick. In particular, the editors would like to thank Sue Dibben and Tracy Horton, who were very helpful at this time, as well as the conference speakers, many of whom contributed to *Picturing Women's Health*. Since then, Tim Lockley (HRC) has continued to provide support, which has been greatly appreciated.

Like the history of women's health, the process of this book has been complex. The editors are especially grateful to Mark Pollard at Pickering & Chatto for his patience and understanding, and would also very much like to thank the contributors, who have stuck with the project and produced some extraordinary work.

Finally, warm thanks are extended to the editors' colleagues, partners, families and friends, who have been generous with their interest, encouragement and enthusiasm.

LIST OF CONTRIBUTORS

Claire Brock is Lecturer in English at the University of Leicester, where she also teaches medical humanities. She has recently completed a monograph entitled *Women Surgeons in Britain, 1860–1918* which was funded by a two-year Research Leave Award from the Wellcome Trust. Other publications include three books, *The Feminization of Fame* (Basingstoke: Palgrave Macmillan, 2006), *The Comet Sweeper* (Thriplow: Icon Books, 2007), and *Victorian Science and Literature* Volume 5, *New Audiences for Science: Women, Children, Labourers* (London: Pickering & Chatto, 2012), as well as a number of recent articles on surgery in the late nineteenth and early twentieth centuries. Her next project is about the experience of the surgical patient in the same period.

Ji Won Chung is a PhD candidate in the Department of English and Comparative Literary Studies at the University of Warwick. Her work focuses on how the late nineteenth-century culture of beauty, fashion and spiritualism Gothicized the female body, along with how such images are represented in the fictions of the period. Her essay, 'Beautiful Monsters: Cosmeticised Women in the Late Victorian Period', is published in L. K. Davis and C. Santos (eds), *The Monster Imagined* (Freeland: Inter-Disciplinary, 2010), pp. 145–58.

Katherine Ford is a PhD candidate working with the University of Reading and the Royal Society on a collaborative project examining the role of the Royal Society in Victorian Literary Culture. Her work focuses on the use of archival resources in examining the relationship of literary and scientific writing for a range of audiences and the interplay of ideas between disciplines, as well as the roles of scientists and literary authors within this landscape.

Alexandra Lewis is Lecturer in English Literature, and Associate Director of the Centre for the Novel, at the University of Aberdeen. She holds a PhD from Trinity College, Cambridge, where she was a Cambridge Commonwealth Trust Scholar. Editor of the *British Association for Victorian Studies Newsletter*, Alexandra serves on the BAVS executive committee. She has taught English Literature at the Universities of London (Goldsmiths), Warwick and several Cambridge colleges. Her research interests include literature and medicine; Neo-Victorian literature; the Brontës; George Eliot; and *fin-de-siècle* psychology. Alexandra's publications on the Brontës include chapters in R. Barnett and S. Trowbridge (eds), *Acts of Memory: The Victorians and Beyond* (Newcastle: Cambridge Scholars Publishing, 2010), pp. 35–53 and in M. Thormählen (ed.), *The Brontës in Context* (Cambridge: Cambridge University Press, 2012), pp. 198–206. She is currently completing a monograph that uncovers an emergent discourse of mental trauma in nineteenth-century literature, culture and psychology.

Andrew McInnes is Lecturer in English (Education and Scholarship) at the University of Exeter, Cornwall Campus. His research focus is on women's writing and Romanticism, particularly political, philosophical and fictional responses to the French Revolution. He has published on Amelia Opie's *Adeline Mowbray*, Mary Hays's *Female Biography*, and feminist polemic at the end of the eighteenth century. He has work forthcoming on women and Gothic, analysing Charlotte Dacre's authorial strategies and reading Jane Austen's continuing engagement with the Gothic, beyond the comic mode of *Northanger Abbey*.

Hilary Marland is Professor of History at the University of Warwick and founder of its Centre for the History of Medicine, which she directed from 1998 to 2009. She is author of *Health and Girlhood in Britain, 1874–1920* (Houndmills: Palgrave Macmillan, 2013) and *Dangerous Motherhood: Insanity and Childbirth in Victorian Britain* (Houndmills: Palgrave Macmillan, 2004). Her research interests span the nineteenth-century medical marketplace, women and mental illness, the history of childbirth and midwifery, migration and mental illness, and household medicine in modern Britain, the topic of her next monograph. She is also developing new work on a major collaborative project on prisons, medicine and human rights in England and Ireland in the modern period.

Joseph Morrissey is a research associate at the University of Warwick and seminar tutor at the University of Manchester. His work explores how the Romantic-period novel presents the interrelations between social space, domestic activity, cognition and emotion.

Sarah Richardson is Associate Professor of History at the University of Warwick. She writes widely on the topic of women and political culture in eighteenth- and nineteenth-century Britain. Her latest monograph is *The Political Worlds of Women: Gender and Political Culture in Nineteenth-Century Britain* (New York: Routledge, 2013).

Kate Scarth is a Postdoctoral Associate Fellow in the Department of English and Comparative Literary Studies at the University of Warwick, where she received her PhD. She is currently working on a monograph on fictional representations of suburban homes in Romantic-period London. Other research interests include Romantic London more generally, critical literary geography, environmental criticism and medical humanities.

Francesca Scott is a lecturer at Amsterdam University College and a postdoctoral researcher at the Huygens ING with the HERA project *Travelling TexTs: The Transnational Reception of Women's Writing at the Fringes of Europe.* She completed her PhD, 'The Fuzzy Theory and Women Writers in the Late Eighteenth Century', at the University of Warwick, and her research interests include women's writing in the long eighteenth century, the history of childbirth, midwifery and women's health, and a number of fields in the medical humanities. Forthcoming publications include *Women Telling Nations* (co-editor, Rodopi, 2014).

Tabitha Sparks is Associate Professor of English at McGill University in Montreal, Canada. She specializes in the nineteenth-century British novel, Victorian cultural studies, literature and medicine, and narrative theory. She is the author of *The Doctor in the Victorian Novel: Family Practices* (Farnham and Burlington, VT: Ashgate, 2009), a collection of nineteenth-century criticism on the Brontës, and numerous essays in journals and book collections. She is currently working on two book projects: one on non-canonical popular Victorian novels, and one on Wilkie Collins.

Susannah Wilson is a British Academy Postdoctoral Research Fellow and Assistant Professor in the Department of French Studies at the University of Warwick. Her postdoctoral research focuses on women, intoxication and self-destruction in nineteenth-century France, analysing medical documents, fiction, art, the press and autobiographical writing by French women. Her research is concerned with the placing of women's voices within contemporary medical discourses about the female body. She is currently writing a monograph on women, opium and morphine in *fin-de-siècle* France.

LIST OF FIGURES

INTRODUCTION: PICTURING WOMEN'S HEALTH

Francesca Scott, Kate Scarth and Ji Won Chung

If a Google images search is any reliable indicator, there are many ways to picture women's health in 2014. A search brings back smiling faces – women, but also men and children of different ages and races from various time periods. These people are in civvies, national costume and medical uniforms; they are sometimes by themselves, other times embracing another person or in some instances surrounded by children or professionals. Women lift weights, exercise and participate in charity runs. Some images show models or drawings of the inside of the human body – the reproductive system or blood cells. Ill health or disease is often implied: in one image, women hold up bras, presumably symbolizing healthy breasts either pre- or post-breast cancer. *Women's Health* magazine, created in 2005 to counterbalance the emphasis on men's bodies in *Men's Health* magazine (founded in 1987), makes several appearances, super buff female bodies gracing its covers. Sometimes there are no people in these images, just food, nature scenes, or graphs, charts or maps pointing to some issue relating to women's health and well-being. The names of clinics also appear, as do cheques representing money made to support them.

These varied images provide a useful introduction to our approach to picturing women's health; this collection broaches many ways of thinking about women's health that move beyond simple or typical notions of 'representing'. A picture can be a 'visual representation', encompassing the graphs, charts and maps referenced above.[1] In this sense, picturing also evokes 'a representation as a work of art', pointing to processes of creation and consumption.[2] In the essays that follow, authors interrogate these methods of picturing female health by considering the artist/creator, the pictured subject, the audience and the explicit aims of the representation; our contributors ask questions such as: what discourses/ideologies/perspectives are implicit/explicit in the work (of art)? What power dynamics are revealed/inherent in such representations? Meanwhile, a picture can also be a 'concrete representation or illustration of an abstract idea or quality; a symbol, type, or figure' or a 'person or thing seen as the embodiment of some quality'.[3] In this way, a smiling face, lush greenery or particular types of food (a fruit smoothie, a pile of grains) represent, illustrate and/or embody (women's) health. Google images provide us with many types of female bodies and ideas about female health (buff, professional, diseased) pictured via various discourses (medical, fitness entertainment, philanthropy). Such variety has long existed: in the nineteenth century, asylum picture, novels and medical journals give us prostitutes, anorexics, angels of the house – bodies that conform, that subvert dominant social structures, bodies that are diseased, that are healthy. Finally, this collection as a whole aims to fulfil another meaning of 'picture': the essays strive to create 'an intellectual model or framework of understanding', to reflect 'a state of affairs', namely that of women's health in the long nineteenth century.[4]

With this approach to picturing, we work alongside other scholars of medical humanities who draw attention to processes of representing, imagining and picturing. For example, Ludmilla Jordanova, in her influential study of gender in biomedical sciences, *Sexual Visions* (1989), states that '[t]he goal of a rich cultural history must be to extend the understanding we derive from social history in order to come to terms with the power of images',[5] while Janis Caldwell analyses nineteenth-century medical and literary texts from a hermeneutic stance in order to 'find ... interpretations that the text's formal properties and cultural embeddedness seem to converge upon'.[6] We specifically take John Wiltshire's framework for analysing health and the body in *Jane Austen and the Body: 'The Picture of Health'* and extend his focus on an early nineteenth-century novelist to a range of genres and documents across the century.[7] Wiltshire's subtitle is drawn from *Emma*, specifically Mrs Weston's appraisal of Emma Woodhouse's health (and beauty) to Mr Knightley:

> 'oh! what a bloom of full health, and such a pretty height and size; such a firm and upright figure! There is health, not merely in her bloom, but in her air, her head, her glance. One hears sometimes of a child being "the picture of health"; now, Emma always gives me the idea of being the complete picture of grown-up health. She is loveliness itself. Mr Knightley, is not she?'[8]

At least two senses of 'picture' can be applied here. Mrs Weston verbally draws a picture of just how healthy Emma is by invoking her physical features and mannerisms – her height, size, air, head, glance – and, as Wiltshire notes, Mrs Weston's words position Emma as an embodiment of health, in other words, she *is* health.[9] Mrs Weston, as Emma's long-time governess and friend, is of course biased here and Mr Knightley, beginning perhaps to realize his true (romantic) feelings for Emma, is an audience willingly held captive to a recitation of her physical virtues. Emma's health is underwritten by her secure socio-economic status which is contrasted, for example, with the ill health of the poor cottagers to whom she delivers broth or even with the less well-off Harriet Smith who suffers from a sore throat and a rotten tooth over the course of the novel. '[H]andsome, clever, and rich', Emma is also largely extracted from larger health debates that are touched on in the novel.[10] While her nervous father and sister debate the relative health merits of the increasingly popular seaside resort towns, Emma only visits the shore for romantic reasons (her honeymoon) rather than for health purposes. Another Austenian 'picture of health' is an even more highly privileged woman – Lady Bertram in *Mansfield Park*: at one point she, 'sunk back in one corner of the sofa, the picture of health, wealth, ease, and tranquillity, was just falling into a gentle doze, while Fanny was getting through the few difficulties of her work for her'.[11] Here Austen paints another picture of what health might look like: a dozing, wealthy lady on a sofa. Lady Bertram embodies health and ease, while her busy niece Fanny is often ill and always at work, emphasizing the power imbalance due to their varying socio-economic statuses and ages. Meanwhile, as Lady Bertram dozes, she fails to act as either mother or regent of Mansfield Park in her husband's absence; during her nap, her children plan the theatrical which their father would stridently oppose as it enables them to act out their illicit romantic and sexual impulses. Lady Bertram's embodiment of health is therefore far from a straightforwardly positive proposition, positioning her as it does as a particular 'type' – namely, a lady of fashion – having every material advantage without putting that wealth or social position to any good purpose. Wider social contexts and various aspects of women's lives are thus bound up with notions of health – broader implications that the essays that follow all consider.

Women's Health in the Period 1770–1910

This complex notion of women's health is evident in, and fully informed by, a wider discourse that included medical treatises, political pamphlets, textbooks and education. One of the participants in this, and perhaps one of the first to fully articulate the relationship between women's health and the wider context of female life, was Mary Wollstonecraft. While the *Vindication of the Rights of Woman* has frequently been reduced to a few pointed remarks about female education, it is as much about exercising the body as it is about exercising female reason and intellect, all with the aim of producing a strong, well-rounded, healthy woman: 'I wish to persuade women to endeavor to acquire strength, both of mind and body'.[12] Indeed, the mind and body are bound together throughout the *Rights of Woman*; rarely does one follow without the other. Wollstonecraft criticizes an education system that sacrifices 'strength of body and mind' to 'libertine notions of beauty', and lambasts an outdated notion of female excellence that makes women proud of delicacy, and 'cramps the activity of the mind'.[13] In her view, 'strength of mind has, in most cases, been accompanied by superior strength of body',[14] and to deny the 'pure animal spirits' that make 'both mind and body shoot out', is to 'contract the faculties and spoil the temper'.[15]

Bodily strength is also tied to sexual character. As Miriam Brody has noted, Wollstonecraft's woman of fashion 'is unable to be virtuous because her body is weak', '"strength of body and mind" are required in the virtuous work of regulating a family, educating children, certainly for the extraordinary work of public writing'.[16] According to Adriana Craciun, this has famously been used to underline Wollstonecraft's 'deep ambivalence about sexuality', but, as Craciun notes, such an interpretation threatens to conflate corporeality with sexuality, when in fact Wollstonecraft offered women much more 'on the subject of the body than warnings about the need to suppress it'.[17] Indeed, if anything, the female body in Wollstonecraft's system is energetic and full of life, her feet are 'eloquent', and her body has acquired 'full vigour',[18] while the way in which girls are 'restrained and cowed', subject to 'wearisome confinement' is sharply criticized.[19] Only by 'bounding, as nature directs', in 'attitudes so conducive to health',[20] can the female body reach its potential, 'preserving health' and 'promoting beauty'.[21]

With this, Wollstonecraft had taken up a thread that her friend and predecessor, Catherine Macaulay, had begun two years previously. In her *Letters on Education with Observations on Religions and Metaphysical Subjects* (1790), Macaulay had also explored the connection between the female body and mind, and had further advocated the Spartan education system as a suitable model for women:

> That the mental powers are affected by an union with corporal weakness; that it commonly gives a taint to the morals; and that conduct uniformly virtuous must be the joint issue of a good head and sound constitution. Bodily strength was the chief object of Spartan discipline. Their cares on this subject began with the birth of their offspring; and instead of entailing feebleness on their women for the sake of augmenting their personal beauty, they endeavoured to improve their natural strength, in order to render them proper nurses for the race of heroes.[22]

Female bodily strength was at the heart of this model, and Macaulay saw the feats of the Spartan women – as warriors – as intrinsic to their ability to bear and nurse healthy children. More than this, she also saw that women had through such exercise the opportunity to escape suppression, and even, ostensibly, their sex and gender: Spartan women were, of course, renowned for their lesbian relationships, a detail of which Macaulay, as an historian, was undoubtedly aware.

The entry of Macaulay and Wollstonecraft into this debate, at such a crucial time in the history of women's health, was no coincidence. The preceding forty or fifty years had seen extraordinary advances in the study of anatomy, particularly in the study of female anatomy, and both writers were almost certainly responding to this. The field was benefiting from increased secularism, and a thirst for detail and accuracy; to see things as they really were, rather than idealized or imagined. That is not to underestimate the influence of the early modern period, however. The period preceding the one outlined in this collection has been recognized as one of extraordinary scientific advancement, of revolution even, and this certainly extends to the field of female medicine and health. Indeed, one might even argue that literature from the early modern period is saturated with references to various aspects of women's health, even at a time when the workings of the female body – and in particular the female reproductive system – were still a relative unknown. The reasons for this were economical; when we talk about women's health, we are often talking about their reproductive health – an emphasis that this collection strives to complicate – and in the early modern period this meant their ability to bear children, and as many as possible, for the benefit of the state. Their ability to conceive quickly, carry healthy babies to full term and then give birth so that they could begin the whole process again was prized, and it made the control of this process all the more important. The effects of this can be observed in the number of midwifery manuals written by women, who can be seen referencing an often unnamed, external threat to their field of work – a new approach – that brought with it the trappings of industry and mechanics: the professionalization of the study of women's reproductive health. Midwives such as Jane Sharp, writing in her *The Midwives Book, Or the Whole Art of Midwifery Discovered* (1671), defended the encroachment, noting that 'women are as fruitful, and as safe and well delivered, if not more fruitful, and better commonly in childbed' than those who are attended by 'Men of Learning'.[23] 'It is not hard words that perform the work', she says, 'words are just the shell'.[24]

By the eighteenth century, at the point at which Wollstonecraft and Macaulay were writing, this tension had intensified, brought about by recent discoveries in anatomy, most famously seen in the work of John and William Hunter, *Anatomia uteri humani gravidi tabulis illustrate* (1774). The engravings by Jan van Rymsdyk from this piece demonstrate an entirely new way of picturing the female body, one that was stripped, literally in the sense that the anatomists removed anything from the frame that was not of interest to the study (including limbs, skin and even hair), and figuratively by deliberately avoiding religious allegory or symbolism. The emphasis was on hard, clinical evidence. It revealed a number of important details about the placenta and maternal blood flow, as well as embryological phases, but the focus, at least in terms of where the eye is drawn in these engravings, is very much on the female genitalia and, in particular, the sectioned clitoris. As Jordanova has argued, there is in this, perhaps, an implicit violence,[25] and certainly something that seeks to divide and conquer the female body.

The significance of such anatomical discoveries has already been extensively interrogated in a number of critical theories, from Thomas Laqueur's one-sex and two-sex theory, to the response of Katharine Park and Robert Nye.[26] The effect that this had specifically in terms of the study of women's health is even more extraordinary; yet, the period has often been overlooked, sandwiched between two apparently more interesting scientific revolutions, that of the fifteenth and sixteenth centuries and of the nineteenth century. In particular, the tension that can be observed between the body, mind, sexuality, health and femininity in the works of Wollstonecraft and Macaulay above, can almost certainly be pinpointed in this period, which stems from the need to control female health, whether by restricting the activity of young women, employing the use of instruments (such as forceps) on childbearing women or encouraging feigned weakness and delicacy as a form of beauty. Such ideas were perpetuated by conduct books, as identified by Wollstonecraft, as well as medical treatises, becoming yet another way of picturing women's health and the female body.

While, then, female health was becoming more properly understood, this did not suggest that women were really feeling the benefit of this; they did not, broadly speaking, have access to new knowledge about their health, or indeed the means of picturing themselves. Moreover, controlling female health – and by extension female sexuality – was crucial. This continued in the nineteenth century, the seat of the second scientific revolution, even as separate disciplines in the sciences emerged, and the emphasis on empirical evidence quickened. By situating *Picturing Women's Health* in a wider social context, it will be shown that discoveries in medicine were now inextricably intertwined with politics, and science was increasingly becoming both the vehicle for emancipation, as well as for control. Acts of Parliament were at the centre of this. Indeed, the Victorian Period is often known as the Age of Reform, and to a large extent it was, with several of these acts directly affecting women: the Factory Act (1833), Mines Act (1842), Matrimonial Causes Act (1857), Contagious Diseases Act (1864) and Married Women's Property Act (1882). It was in this period that the issue of women's health was thrust into the public sphere, becoming widely accepted as an issue that had far-reaching consequences.

The Contagious Diseases Act was one such act to be directly aimed at the issue of health, and, as a system of regulating prostitution, aimed specifically at women. It gave policemen the power to spy on and retain any woman they suspected of being a prostitute, and subject her to an internal examination. If she was found to have a disease, such as gonorrhea or syphilis, she could be interred in a Lock Hospital, a clinic that specialized in venereal disease, for up to nine months, and thereafter receive fortnightly internal inspections. Not surprisingly, this often meant that women of a lower class, particularly if they were found in a military town, were forced to undergo a traumatic examination without any evidence that they were indeed prostitutes, while men escaped any kind of examination or sanction. In response, women such as Josephine Butler, an early feminist and campaigner, began a repeal campaign, arguing that the Contagious

Diseases Act was unjust in that it 'unpunished the sex [i.e. men] who are the main cause, both of the vice and of its dreaded consequences'.[27] The act highlighted the disparity between the way in which the health of men and women was viewed: the protection and stability of men's health was paramount, while prostitutes were, as Mavis Kirkham has argued, seen 'simply as containers of infection', and could, as such, be subject to censure and violation.[28] It also underlined class distinction and an officially sanctioned double standard of sexual morality, noted by Judith R. Walkowitz.[29] More importantly, it relied on a notion that women could not be seen as anything other than patients. There was yet little room for autonomy, and even less for women to take charge of their sphere of health, as practitioners, although some were (and had even before this period) defied this.

While men were prying into the female body, they were also prying into the female mind. The interrogation of the mind–body binary had not lost any of its urgency in the proceeding sixty or seventy years since Wollstonecraft's *Rights of Woman*, but had, quite conversely, been even further problematized. Those operating within the medical sphere, and particularly in the emerging sphere of psychology, indeed saw that the two were inextricable, but rather than seeing the mind as benefiting from a healthy body, one that is active and allowed to bloom, as Wollstonecraft and Macaulay had, they instead saw the female body as a threat. At the centre of this was, as before, the female reproductive system. As Laurence Talairach-Vielmas has explored, the functions of the female reproductive system were 'associated with an array of nervous disorders which justified medical surveillance', and as a result, middle-class women were defined as 'frail, unstable, and governed by their reproductive functions',[30] inseparable from their biology. In this collection, Hilary Marland notes that this was indicative of a preoccupation with menstruation, a seemingly inexplicable process that seemed to be an excess of the female body. It was not until the 1860s that medicine confirmed that menstruation was dependent on the ovaries, and even then the medical field continued to regard it with suspicion.[31] As Sally Shuttleworth explains, this became an 'obsessive focus for the male imagination, symbolizing, with its bloody, uncontrollable flow, the dark otherness of woman'.[32] Scholars have persuasively argued that this has been pictured in a variety of novels from the period, including, for instance, Bram Stoker's *Dracula* (1897).[33] Likewise, medical treatises explored the apparent correlation between menstruation and insanity, noting countless instances where women had experienced psychotic episodes and had even been driven to murder, brought about at various stages of the menstrual cycle. This thereby demonstrates that women's health could be pictured in ways that were skewed or opaque. As such, Mary Jacobus, Evelyn Fox Keller and Sally Shuttleworth explain that the threat of insanity 'loomed large' in the Victorian era, becoming almost the 'determining condition of womanhood'.[34] This fascination left women vulnerable to accusations of insanity, and meant that they could be locked away (in much the same way as they could be locked away in Lock Hospitals for venereal disease), for doubtful reasons, based on flimsy evidence. Famous novels exploring this include, of course, Wilkie Collins's *The Woman in White* (1859) and Charlotte Brontë's *Jane Eyre* (1847). Both can be seen to be as much about masculine fear and anxiety, as they are about feminine insanity. They also demonstrate the way in which these advances and struggles were being pictured in a variety of different genres, undoubtedly promoted by a new debate exploring the consilience between literature and science, and articulated concretely for the first time by Matthew Arnold in this period.[35]

This unbalanced preoccupation with 'looking within' female nature, as Andrew Mangham has called it,[36] both physically and psychologically, demonstrates that the study of women's health had re-established the complex mind–body dualism that was now very much about control, and particularly about containment. Nineteenth-century medical practices were bent on 'securing gender spheres and controlling female autonomy', while the body was 'harness[ed] and tam[ed]'.[37] Moreover, as this collection will show, women were forced into an ill-fitting frame that pictured them, and their health, in an unflattering (and even harmful) hue. In particular, it perpetuated the image of the female invalid, a role that was fully endorsed in nineteenth-century Britain,[38] and supported by the medical profession.[39] It was, ultimately, the physician who decided if the woman was healthy or unhealthy. The power relationship between the woman and her physician was indeed particularly problematic. According to Lorna Duffin, the medical theories and treatments for women were specifically designed with the aim to justify social control, with a number of these treatments seeming especially cruel and barbaric.[40] They included applying leaches to the cervix or uterus, or even surgical procedures, such as clitoridectomy. The outcome of this treatment was, of course, that a number of women suffered injuries that seriously impaired their health. Recovery from such procedures could take months, and may even have affected them for the rest of their lives. On occasion they were even fatal. Not surprisingly, this exacerbated the fear around women's health, the sense of which (as well as the movement to oppose it) can be observed in a number of chapters throughout the collection. In particular, it prevented women from seeking help for serious medical complaints, often until it was too late. The paradox was, as Shirley Roberts has correctly identified, that the Victorians emphasized feminine modesty, and yet women were required to consult *male* physicians.[41]

As can be seen with the campaign around the Contagious Diseases Act, this was increasingly met with opposition from women themselves, who were seeking to take control, to understand their bodies and its associated processes. In the suffragette movement, noted by Sarah Richardson in this collection, this came with self-starvation, a way of achieving autonomy, bodily and politically, against an oppressive state. Force-feeding only underscored what women, according to Lisa Appignanes, already felt: 'reduced to body, even that body wasn't ultimately their own'.[42] Other women were seeking to assume control by entering the professions associated with women's health. Indeed, the period covered by *Picturing Women's Health* ends with a new stage, covered by Claire Brock, in the history of women's health: the entry of women, en masse, into the profession, as nurses, doctors and surgeons, initially to treat other women – to address a need. The power dynamics seen here extended to many other spheres in the context of women's health, from general employment to education and fashion. The image of the female patient, while still conspicuous for many decades, was steadily being replaced with the vision of the female doctor, with skill, courage and a strong constitution. It is, perhaps, the most obvious way in which women's health affected women's social and professional status: once women had broken through this barrier, others soon fell, and the sphere of women's health could encompass images of woman in diverse roles, not merely as mother, wife, prostitute and patient. Crucially, this had the effect of breaking open, and bringing new meaning to, the mind–body dualism, which could now incorporate female reason for the first time – as had been astutely and prophetically pictured by Wollstonecraft nearly one hundred and fifty years previously.

Picturing Women's Health thus seeks to enrich our understandings of women's health in a few key ways. Much work has considered women's health in terms of female-specific concerns, such as childbirth, menstruation and hysteria.[43] Alternatively, scholars consider a specific type or group of women, such as in recent work on female medical practitioners in the Victorian period.[44] There is also a plethora of scholarship on 'the Victorian body' and 'the female body' and much of this focuses on sexual and gendered power relations in scientific and medical discourses. As Roger Cooter points out, 'corporeality and pathology have become obligatory points of passage in the study of Victorian society and culture'.[45]

The essays that follow engage with these ideas, while complicating them in various ways. The collection as a whole does not just investigate illnesses that were considered peculiar to women, nor does it simply read the body as a historical text, a move which, as Cooter argues, maintains 'reductive methodology and ... reductive biological categories'.[46] Instead, the essays investigate women's varied relationships to both good *and* ill health in the context of their multifaceted and complex lives. Furthermore, rather than thinking about women as a collective, we consider women's individuality and diversity in terms of factors like socio-economic status, profession and lifestyle.

Our authors thus picture many women, types of (ill)health, social contexts and sources. Joseph Morrissey considers the intersection of health, sensibility and financial security in Charlotte Smith's novel *Ethelinde* (1798). Andrew McInnes also looks at a Romantic-period novel – Maria Edgeworth's *Belinda* (1801)

– in the context of other representations, namely James Gillray's satirical visual caricatures, to examine notions of fashion, naturalness and health in relation to women's bodies and social roles. As the nineteenth century progressed, women increasingly took on formal, professional and/or public roles in the world of medicine and health. Sarah Richardson examines women's increasingly public podium in her discussion of how women's rights activists linked feminism, public health and national politics in the late nineteenth century. Meanwhile, Alexandra Lewis investigates the particular generic challenges inherent in fiction's representation of mental illness before turning to the link between theories of miasma and traumatic mental suffering in Charlotte Brontë's *Villette* (1853). We then turn to Susannah Wilson, who explores the iconography of anorexia from 1873–1914 when it emerged as a distinctly modern disease. Tabitha Sparks examines the memoirs of a travelling nurse, Kate Marsden, to explore the picture she painted of herself as a woman who was doubly exposed to the dangers of a contagious disease – leprosy – and to public criticism. Katherine Ford takes us inside the Lawn Hospital in Lincoln giving us detailed readings of clinical photographs in order to complicate typical associations of Victorian mental illness with femininity. Claire Brock's essay offers insight into the many social, physical, mental and professional pressures on female medical students at the turn of the twentieth century. Finally, Hilary Marland provides a picture of popular and medical approaches to adolescent girls' health and well-being. In all, we hope that these essays' approaches to picturing will help create a more wholistic 'model' or 'framework' for approaching representations of women's health and well-being in the long nineteenth century, and that our varied and interdisciplinary approaches forge new links, ripe for future study.

1 SENSIBILITY AND GOOD HEALTH IN CHARLOTTE SMITH'S *ETHELINDE*

Joseph Morrissey

> There are as many and as different Degrees of *Sensibility* or *Feeling* as there are Degrees of *Intelligence* and Perception in *human* Creatures; and the *Principle* of both may be perhaps one and the same. One shall suffer more from the Prick of a *Pin*, or *Needle*, from their extreme Sensibility, than others from being run thro' the Body; and the *first* sort, seem to be of the *Class* of these *Quick-Thinkers* I have formerly mentioned; and as none have it in their *Option* to choose for themselves their own particular *Frame* of Mind nor *Constitution* of Body; so none can choose *his* own Degree of *Sensibility*.[1]

This is one definition of the popular theory of 'sensibility' as offered by Dr George Cheyne, doctor to Samuel Richardson. Eighteenth-century understandings of health were heavily influenced by sensibility. Grounded in influential works by John Locke, Isaac Newton, David Hume and Adam Smith among others, the idea of sensibility was based upon a conception of the elasticity of the nervous system. The link between 'quick-thinkers' and those susceptible to physical pain posits a link between sensitivity of mind and sensitivity of body, a current of thought common to much writing on sensibility in the period. In the privileged classes with access to luxury goods, the excessive consumption of fine food and drink was considered a threat to the constitution, and particularly to the constitution of those with great sensibility. Equally, the sensitive feeling of mind associated with those of sensibility was thought to render them vulnerable to nervous disorders caused by acute emotional distress. Unsurprisingly, perhaps, as the eighteenth century progressed the concept of sensibility was used to delineate gender difference. G. J. Barker-Benfield notes that '[i]n the last third of the [eighteenth] century, "tenderness" became synonymous with sensibility as a characteristic of women',[2] and other words such as 'delicacy' and 'delicate' were increasingly used to denote a particularly feminine state of the nerves which were seen as inherently more sensitive – and therefore more susceptible to disorder – than the nerves of men in the Romantic period. *Ethelinde* (1789) intervenes into this conception of a Romantic-period, feminized sensibility which I take as a key idea which informs my reading of Smith's novel and the surprising perspective on women's health it offers.

Exploring women's sensibility became a staple of the novel in the Romantic period, ranging from depictions in Austen's now famous *Sense and Sensibility* (1811) to those in a host of lesser-known works in which the feeling and delicacy of women is of paramount importance. *Ethelinde* is one such novel, but in rehearsing a well-known theme of the Romantic-period novel the text subjects the theory of sensibility to a subtle critique. Austen's *Sense and Sensibility* at least in part engages with a contemporary debate which points to the selfishness that self-indulgent feeling could lead to. Smith's novel, by contrast, emphasizes the empathy made possible by powerful feelings which permit one to experience the pains of another more acutely. In a radical turn, however, Smith argues that it is precisely the ability to emphasize which allows one to mistreat others for self-interested motives: *Ethelinde* argues that feeling for others represents the most effective method for manipulating and exploiting them.

Smith achieves this perspective on sensibility through the specific narrative style in which *Ethelinde* is presented, and this is a style which resists current interpretations of the development of the novel in the period. Experimentation and refinement of narrative voice was widespread in the late eighteenth- and early nineteenth-century novel. In this collection, Andrew McInnes shows how in *Belinda* (1801) Maria Edgeworth weaves a web of intertextual references through third-person narration to add additional levels of meaning to the text. Edgeworth experimented too with unreliable first-person narration in *Castle Rackrent* (1800). Marilyn Butler's seminal *Jane Austen and the War of Ideas* (1975) emphasized the achievement of technical excellence in third-person narrative voice through free indirect discourse in the novels of Jane Austen. More recently, critics have traced the emergence of free indirect discourse to earlier novelists, and highlighted Austen's debt to her predecessors. Jane Spencer, for example, writes that Frances Burney's development of third-person narration in *Cecilia* is a 'style, in which the third-person narrative takes on a colouring from the characters' idiom and consciousness',[3] and that Burney was a 'pioneer'[4] of free indirect discourse. Spencer continues that Austen's 'free indirect style is much more flexible than Burney's, consistently achieving a combination of sympathy and subtle irony which Burney reaches only occasionally, but Austen's debt to the older novelist is considerable'.[5] Apparent in Spencer's remarks is the construction of a lineage of third-person narration closely tied to the development of free indirect discourse, and that technical perfection in third-person narration is closely aligned with technical perfection in free indirect discourse. Smith's narrator in *Ethelinde*, I will argue, cannot be productively understood within this critical framework. It is precisely the relative absence of free indirect discourse within third-person narration, I will explain, that permits Smith to create a unique perspective on women's health.

I will explore Smith's original approach by considering how the text is pictured through three distinct levels of the reading experience. First there is the story itself. This consists of the events of the story which are given as fact within the fictional framework of the text. The events of the story cannot be evaluated purely objectively: the causal relationship of events which constitutes the plot encourages certain perspectives on the text at the expense of others. To take an example from Jane Austen, in *Mansfield Park* Sir Thomas Bertram is stern and displeased when he learns that Fanny intends to refuse Henry Crawford's proposal of marriage. Because the reader is privy to Henry Crawford's moral failings and understands Fanny is in love Edmund Bertram (both unbeknownst to Sir Thomas), Sir Thomas's severity will tend to appear in more negative light than it might if the story were not structured in this way. Objective reflection may or may not conclude that Sir Thomas is unduly severe, but, crucially, purely objective reflection is impossible in the reading experience. The reader's knowledge of Fanny's private feelings and Henry Crawford's dubious character increases sympathy for Fanny when Sir Thomas forcefully urges her to marry Henry and simultaneously increases the reader's displeasure at Sir Thomas, who becomes the villain in the sequence despite the fact he is denied the facts that might make him act differently. Of course, readers are not mere slaves to emotive impressions, and may take this into account, but nevertheless the unfolding of the events of the story encourage disdain of Sir Thomas's behaviour on a rhetorical, emotive and subjective level. Story structure, of course, is created at the extra-textual level of authorship, and the author therefore has a large degree of control over how characters are perceived according to the specificity of the plot. Within the framework of the text itself, however, the events of the story are given as fact, and any manipulation of reader opinion caused by their organization cannot be attributed to the language or tone of the narrator but only to the seemingly arbitrary unfolding of events.

The second level is the narration of the story, which is rendered in the third person in *Ethelinde*. As already stated, free indirect discourse is very limited in *Ethelinde*, if apparent at all. When Ethelinde's thoughts and feelings are presented, the narrator is always external to them, creating the sense of the narrator as a limited observer of the story even as he/she also tells the story. This is in contrast to free indirect discourse in which the narrator is able to slip into the internal thought and feeling processes of the text's characters so as to become one with them, appearing as a god-like entity that moves ethereally and authoritatively through the text. Equally, the capacity of free indirect discourse to offer subtle ironic commentary on the thoughts and feelings of the presented characters enforces the sense of the narrator's omniscience and authority. With the deft use of free indirect discourse narration of the story becomes inseparable from the story itself, the narrator appearing to some degree *as part of the story's construction* rather than as its mere watcher and teller. The relative absence of omniscience in Smith's narrator opens up a series of questions: is the narrator's interpretation correct? Does the narrator have a motive? Is the narrator trustworthy? In *Ethelinde*, it becomes increasingly apparent that the narrator is untrustworthy and is always attempting to report the story to show the eponymous heroine to advantage, and this makes 'reading' the narrator a central concern of reading *Ethelinde*.

The absence of free indirect discourse in *Ethelinde* encourages interrogation of the limited perspective of the narrative voice, but the absence of free indirect discourse does not in itself guarantee that the reader interrogates the narrator's interpretation of the story. In Edgeworth's *Belinda*, for example, in which the application of free indirect discourse is limited, the unquestioned authority of the narrative voice in the text nevertheless creates a sense of the narrator's omniscience. Because, in *Belinda*, the narrator is presented as a reliable, transparent medium for expressing the truth of the story as it is distilled from the facts of the story, the reader is encouraged to trust the narrator's perspective. In *Ethelinde*, the absence of free indirect discourse is the precondition that enables the unreliability of the narrative voice, but it is only the growing awareness of this unreliability – which is made possible by the interpretative space existing between the three levels of the story – which encourages an incredulous approach to the narrative voice. Unreliable narration is characteristic of texts in the first person, but first-person narration would not allow Smith to produce the perspective on women's health she achieves in *Ethelinde*. The ability of third-person narration to give insight into character thought and feeling processes is vital to Smith's elucidation of the theory of sensibility and its implications for women's health. Equally, the bias and misreading of Smith's narrator are vital in exposing the theory of sensibility to a subtle critique. In short, Smith's picture of women's health is entirely dependent on the specific narrative style she employs.

The final level of the representation comes from the actions of Ethelinde herself. Although Ethelinde's story can ultimately only be related by the narrator, Ethelinde's actions cannot be reduced to the narrator's perspective. Ethelinde's actions within the text are part of the (fictional) facts of the story, the sense of her individual agency highlighted by the narrator's limited perspective and relative distance from Ethelinde, in contrast to texts that feature free indirect discourse heavily and which tend to blur the clear line between characterization and the narration of the story by implicating the narrator in the thought and feeling processes of the presented characters. In *Ethelinde*, when the narrator chooses to focus on certain aspects of the story while sidelining others, when language and imagery are exploited to create a certain tone, we can say that the narrator is spinning the action, but this manipulation does not extend to creating Ethelinde's actions themselves. At the level of the text, Ethelinde is an autonomous being who acts as she wishes beyond the control of the narrator.

Turning now to women's health in *Ethelinde*, I focus on Ethelinde's struggle for monetary, emotional and romantic fulfilment and the implications for health this struggle puts into motion. Financial (in)stability is of significant concern to Ethelinde. Her slender inheritance has been lost because of the gambling habits of her brother, Harry Chesterville, and to a lesser extent of her father, Colonel Chesterville. Both Harry and Colonel Chesterville may be considered to have 'elastic nerves'. The Colonel, for example, 'felt every moment's reflection on the present situation of his children encrease the anguish of his mind and diminish the strength of his body',[6] which explicitly links the Colonel's difficult circumstances to his emotional and physical health. Of Harry, we are told he was 'one of those characters which feel acutely, but only for a moment; and whose temper, equally thoughtless and sanguine, never considers consequences, or despairs of evading them'.[7] In Harry, therefore, elastic nerves do not produce empathy for others, but his capacity to feel powerfully nevertheless points to a state of high sensibility. The health implications of the sensibility of these two characters are brought to the fore when Harry is taken to debtor's prison and becomes so desperate he contemplates suicide, aligning financial stability with psychological (ill-)health and the spectre of ultimate self-violence. Colonel Chesterville, overcome by the severity of his family's financial situation, contracts a fatal physical illness, directly tying a lack of money to physical decay.

Ethelinde's need for financial security also takes on an explicit dimension of health. Complicating her struggle for financial stability is her love for the text's hero, Montgomery. Since he is an impoverished gentleman surviving on his mother's limited funds, marriage to Montgomery would be further detrimental to Ethelinde's already precarious financial situation. As such, Ethelinde refuses to marry Montgomery until their finances are secure. Equally, however, Ethelinde's powerful feelings for Montgomery at once point to a state of high sensibility and allude to serious emotional – and as a consequence possible serious physical – symptoms should she be frustrated in marrying the man she loves. In order to facilitate a prudent marriage to Montgomery, Ethelinde exploits the monetary, social and emotional resources of her cousin by marriage, Sir Edward Newenden. She is able to do this because Sir Edward, despite being married to Ethelinde's cousin Lady Newenden, is deeply in love with Ethelinde and is willing to go to great lengths for her benefit. As the story progresses, it becomes increasingly apparent that Ethelinde is aware of Sir Edward's feelings, and that she deliberately exploits them for her own benefit. Ethelinde's manipulative tendencies, however, are not transparent in the reading experience. Ethelinde is indeed possessed of great sensibility: she relentlessly attends to her brother in debtor's prison, selling all she can to alleviate his financial distress, and staying with him for emotional support even as her own health suffers as a result. Indeed, Ethelinde becomes herself dangerously ill after tending to Sir Edward's seriously sick and contagious child with little rest or sustenance. Apparent throughout the text is Etehlinde's genuine sympathy for others and willingness to suffer them. Moreover, Ethelinde's character is contrasted with the affected emotional lives of the other female characters, including the vain and selfish Lady Newenden, who pretends to faint in order to get male attention; with Ethelinde's other cousin Clarinthia Ludford who apes the excessive sensibility of the heroines in the novels she loves to read despite actually, possessing little in the way of feeling; and with Lady Arabella, who disguises her true cold and ambitious character beneath a veil of acted modesty and sensitivity. Rehearsing a staple of Romantic-period literature, the deeply feeling heroine of sensibility, Ethelinde, embodies true sensitivity of feeling in contrast to these female characters who feign and exploit ideas of sensibility for their own gain, with the result that Ethelinde's self-interested behaviour becomes difficult to recognize. In stark contrast to the authentic heroine of sensibility, however, Ethelinde actually uses her highly sensitive and empathetic nature for her own gains. To be clear, I am not trying to situate *Ethelinde* within a context of conservative and anti-Jacobin literature that understands powerful internal feelings as self-indulgent and ultimately selfish.[8] In the text, this type of feeling is represented by the more marginal Harry Chesterville, whose self-indulgent feeling only clarifies the rather different ways of feeling characteristic of Ethelinde. In a surprising move, *Ethelinde* understands sensitivity towards others, empathy and truly selfless feeling as being ultimately selfish.

The text's representation of Ethelinde's relationship with her would-be suitor, a vain and ignorant young gentleman by the name of Davenant, provides insight into Smith's narratological strategy in the context of the three levels of the text outlined above. Ethelinde is caught outside at night in a thunderstorm far from her lodgings, and alarmed by the sight of a fisherman (who is in fact Montgomery), is relieved to find his manners mark him as a gentleman and that he is extremely handsome; she is therefore pleased to accept his proposal to escort her to safety. A few days later, Montgomery saves Ethelinde from drowning. Ethelinde is still unconscious when Montgomery leaves her to the care of her relatives, but the universal report of the handsome stranger's bravery strongly arouses Ethelinde's curiosity. Davenant accompanies Ethelinde on a walk, and upon seeing Montgomery's cottage, Ethelinde had 'in a few moments ... argued herself into the most perfect conviction of the propriety of what she was desirous to do, and pursued the path which led to the cottage'.[9] Davenant objects:

> 'Why should you visit this young man?' said he. 'I do not believe he is a person of consequence enough to make it necessary. Besides, I should think it not quite correct: had you not better write to thank him, and all that sort of thing?'[10]

According to prevalent social conventions in the period, Davenant is entirely correct here, since a respectable lady would not ordinarily pay personal respects to a fisherman stranger whose social connections were unknown. Moreover, without a proper introduction it would be considered improper to simply come to his residence: Ethelinde should indeed 'write ... and all that sort of thing'. These are the facts of the story, but they are rendered unstable by both the specific plotting of the events, and also by Ethelinde herself. First, Davenant's use of the phrase 'all that sort of thing' reflects a fashionable style of speech, evoking his close connections to elite metropolitan culture and thus to a class of people whose dissipated tendencies were frequently perceived as immoral in the period, and which certainly are perceived this way within the overall context of *Ethelinde*, which ultimately endorses values of economy, quiet living and modesty. As such, Davenant's style of speech immediately associates him with immorality. Moreover, imprecise speech was a symptomatic device in the period to suggest moral failings: how can one really understand proper codes of behaviour if one cannot even articulate them? The point is further driven home by Ethelinde's response: '"That sort of thing", answered Ethelinde, smiling, "is not the sort of thing that appears sufficiently expressive of my gratitude towards the man who saved my life"'.[11]

Ethelinde clearly articulates the specifics of her connection with Montgomery in contrast to Davenant's vague reference to social convention. Moreover, Ethelinde's gentle witticism against Davenant lends her remarks a rhetorical power which will tend to engage the reader with her at the expense of Davenant. Further, before Davenant makes his correct statement concerning social convention, he rather abruptly asks 'Why should you visit this man?',[12] and points out Montgomery's low 'consequence'.[13] Although Davenant's observations are correct, his blunt reference to Montgomery's social rank is indelicate, and prefigures the malicious jealousy of Montgomery which will soon become the principle aspect of Davenant's personality, and which retrospectively casts further doubt over his thinking in this instance. The plotting of events, which juxtaposes Ethelinde with Davenant at the moment of her indiscretion, therefore works to mask her impropriety. Equally, Ethelinde herself is implicated in this rhetorical effect since it is heavily determined by the wit, precision and gentility of her words relative to Davenant. Moreover, by gesturing towards the circumstances that led to Montgomery saving her life, Ethelinde invokes an emotive rhetoric which works to lessen the sense of her actions' impropriety, disabling objective reason under emotive power. This analysis on the novel itself demonstrates quite clearly how the levels of the text can function in creating an objectively unstable perception of Ethelinde and her actions.

Ethelinde refuses Davenant's proposal of marriage despite Sir Edward urging the alliance (primarily because Davenant is wealthy). In terms of health,

Ethelinde is wise to refuse Davenant. Davenant's financial stability is a chimera because his gambling addiction is always threatening ruin and thus the well-being of any future wife (gambling, after all, leads to the nervous disorders that cause Colonel Chesterville's death). Moreover, sensibility, and especially *female* sensibility, was understood to predispose the individual to nervous disorders caused by ill-manners, as expressed by Samuel Richarsdon's Lovelace: 'A man that is gross in a woman's company ought to be knocked down with a club, for, like so many musical instruments, touch but a single wire, and the dear souls are sensible all over'.[14]

In this respect, marriage to Davenant would be detrimental to Ethelinde's health because, for example, he becomes 'thoroughly sulky'[15] when a light-hearted joke is made at his expense, and receives it 'with very ill grace',[16] illustrating his symptomatic immature and ill-bred social behaviour. Even worse, Davenant becomes progressively more malicious in his actions as the story progresses, culminating in a violent attempt to make Ethelinde his mistress, which almost results in rape. Most significantly, perhaps, Davenant's links with elite metropolitan culture are unsuited to Ethelinde's more retired genteel tastes. Davenant is taken under the tutelage of the dastardly Lord Danesforte, a man 'who piqued himself on the deepest politics',[17] and whose 'houses, his equipages, his horses, his mistresses, his dinners, were the theme of the day',[18] and thereby introduced into a fashionable aristocratic lifestyle valuing self-display, self-will and conspicuous consumption. Ethelinde is frequently exasperated and exhausted by the brash company of Danesforte and Davenant, such as when she 'was by no means able to answer ... [the] trifling raillery'[19] of Danesforte, and was in fact 'near to shedding tears'[20] because of his insensitive remarks, pointing to how marrying into such a culture would likely have a detrimental effect on her nerves. Moreover, Danesforte prides himself on being able to 'drink a great deal'[21] and Davenant gradually descends into alcoholism as the story progresses. Since, as stated in the introduction to this chapter, nervous disorders were understood to arise from excessive consumption as well as from emotional distress, the heavy drinking associated with elite urban culture is especially unhealthy for a person of sensibility (such as Ethelinde).

Ethelinde's refusal of Davenant's proposal is in the interest of long-term health and seems entirely understandable within the overall context of the text. At the minutiae level of narrative description, however, a less savoury view of Ethelinde is apparent. Ethelinde uses Sir Edward as a 'middle-man' between Davanent and herself, manipulating the former into rejecting Davenant in her place, so as to save her an uncomfortable encounter. The narrative representation of this, however, works towards the mystification of Ethelinde's selfishness. Initially, Ethelinde tells Sir Edward that should Davenant wish to know her reasons for refusal, she should give them to him. Later on the same day, Sir Edward raises the subject of Davenant again:

> 'What am I to say to Davenant? He complains that he has in vain sought an opportunity of speaking to you; that you repulse him without hearing him; and he has been asking me if I will allow him to escort you part of the way to-morrow, that he may have an opportunity of explaining himself'.
>
> 'I hope, Sir, you refused him?'
>
> 'I referred him to you'.
>
> 'I am sorry that you did, because it puts me to the pain of rejecting peremptorily a mark of attention, for which I am doubtless obliged to Mr. Davenant, but which I can by means accept'.
>
> 'Suffer him then to speak to you this evening, and let him hear your resolution from yourself. May I tell him that you will hear him?'[22]

Despite having earlier stated she would give Davenant reasons for her refusal should he so request, she now wishes to avoid doing so. Moreover, by placing the emphasis on her own discomfort (that it would be unpleasant for her to have to tell Davenant she does not wish to marry him), she forgets Davenant might suffer; furthermore, she forgets or ignores the difficult situation she forces Sir Edward into by using him to handle Davenant. Finally, since Sir Edward is in love with Ethelinde, and since she knows this, her appeal to her own uneasiness is a clear attempt at manipulating Sir Edward to do her bidding, since she is aware that 'deprived of almost all other happiness, [Sir Edward] found his greatest consolation in contributing to the ease and relief of Ethelinde'.[23] Ethelinde's exploitation of Sir Edward's affections is seen most clearly when she says 'if you have indeed the affection for me which I have always been so proud of, persuade him [Davenant] to desist from a pursuit which persecutes and perplexes me'.[24] Implying that Sir Edward cannot really feel for Ethelinde if he does not do as she wishes, this emotionally loaded statement is an unashamed play upon Sir Edward's feelings of guilt. Ethelinde does not act without empathy, however: I have given evidence to demonstrate Etehlinde's strong attachment to Sir Edward, and her genuine concern for his well-being in the introduction to this chapter, and it is a point repeatedly made apparent by the facts of the story, the narrator, and by Ethelinde herself. It is precisely Ethelinde's strong sensibility which allows her to connect with Sir Edward's feelings in powerful ways, and therefore exploit him. The seemingly passive state of feeling acutely is reworked into a proactive social strategy. In parallel with the text's characters who forcefully follow their own will within the context of dissipation and libertinism, and with the female characters who affect sensibility for self-interested motives, the condition of acute sensibility can be used as an aggressive social strategy aimed at self-satisfaction, often to the detriment of others.

Despite these failings of decency on Ethelinde's part, however, a causal reading likely invites sympathy. In the passage examined above, Ethelinde graciously acknowledges her gratitude to Davenant for his favour, enforcing the impression of her good breeding, and the reader's knowledge of Davenant's multiple faults will tend to create sympathy with the text's heroine rather than her inferior would-be suitor. A combination of Ethelinde's own actions and the structure of events, therefore, combine in Ethelinde's favour. This passage follows immediately after Sir Edward has entreated Ethelinde to see Davenant the second time:

> This was almost too much for Ethelinde; who, overcome by the pain of having parted for ever from the man who possessed her heart, was yet compelled to listen to proposals from another, for whom she felt only indifference bordering on contempt; and whom she found herself disposed to dislike the more, because he possessed all those pecuniary advantages, the want of which in Montgomery deprived her of all hope of being his.[25]

By emphasizing Ethelinde's acute feeling and emotional pain, this passage works to create sympathy with Ethelinde, and thereby tends to mask her indiscretions. Ethelinde herself is partly responsible since it is she who experiences powerful romantic feelings for Montgomery. Moreover, because Ethelinde's feelings for Montgomery are explicitly formulated in tandem with those she has for Davenant, and because her love for Montgomery increases her dislike of Davenant, the reader's sympathy with Ethelinde becomes inseparable from the reader's aversion to Davenant, further mitigating the sense of Ethelinde's ill-treatment of him. Although it is Ethelinde who feels these reported sensations, it is the narrator's decision to represent them in detail and in an emotive style. The narrator is therefore also implicated in helping to mask the self-will and ill-treatment of others inherent in Ethelinde's application of sensibility.

The story is also structured to Ethelinde's advantage because it highlights her conformity to contemporary ideals of feminine gentility. Since women were seen as inherently more sensible, the theory of sensibility supported the existing patriarchal mode of production in which the father/husband was culturally and legally the head of the household. Men's supposedly more controlled emotions and their greater rationality enable them to protect women from excessive emotions and nervous disorders.[26] In light of this, the text's presentation of the relationship between Ethelinde and Davenant takes on particular cultural significance. Davenant's proposal comes amidst the news that Ethelinde's father is in distress, and that he requires her immediate return. Ethelinde asks Sir Edward why they should waste time talking of Davenant 'when my heart is with my father, and I am impatient to follow?'[27] So impatient, in fact, that she implores Sir Edward to '[c]ontrive it for me ... so that I may lose no more time',[28] that she may 'prepare instantly for ... departure'.[29] This is in spite of the fact that she must leave her lover, Montgomery, 'who she was perhaps never to see again!'[30] Ethelinde's powerful feelings for Montgomery denote her feminine sensibility, but she will not let this stand in the way of her love and duty to her father, and as such she emerges as the perfect distillation of an ideal feminine gentility. The story is worked so these ideals are brought to the fore during Ethelinde's treatment of the Davenant proposal, and in this context her handling of Sir Edward and Davenant is likely to appear understandable, even heroic, in spite of its underlying failings of decency.

In order to continue to exploit the financial support of Sir Edward, Ethelinde must ensure that his romantic feelings for her remain strong. This, however, risks causing jealousy and resentment in Montgomery. Montgomery treats the sensitive subject of Sir Edward's feelings for Ethelinde with respect, delicately suggesting that Sir Edward probably did not think 'of the danger till it was not to be escaped',[31] a point validated early in the story when it is stated that Ethelinde's company 'instilled into his [Sir Edward's] heart a slow secret poison, which he detected not till it was no longer in his power to expel it'.[32] Similarly, Montgomery claims that the 'misconduct of his [Sir Edward's] wife helped, while it put all your [Ethelinde's] perfections in too striking contrast',[33] another point validated repeatedly, such as when the reader is told that Sir Edward had 'caught himself making involuntary comparisons between her [Ethelinde] and his wife'.[34] Moreover, Montgomery tentatively suggests that Lady Newenden's errors are 'not to the extent which has been represented'.[35] This is also correct: Lady Newenden has in reality done nothing worse than flirt with the libertine Lord Danesforte, and this is at least partly in response to Sir Edward's persistently inappropriate behaviour towards Ethelinde. Finally, Montgomery states that 'nothing can persuade me that in pursuing a divorce Sir Edward has not in contemplation a future and more happy union',[36] an assertion borne out by the fact that Sir Edward does propose to Ethelinde once he believes it is possible she might accept him. Ethelinde responds as follows to Montgomery's take on Sir Edward's one-sided lover affair:

> 'Gracious God!' cried Ethelinde, bursting into a flood of tears, 'is it then certain that you – that Montgomery can join with the malicious, the invidious world, in imputing the most generous actions to the most unworthy motives? ... this shall be our last conference on the subject'.[37]

Montgomery's sensitive, measured speech is very far from 'joining the malicious world'[38] and 'imputing the most generous actions to the most unworthy motives'.[39] Ethelinde employs highly emotive and hyperbolic language to carry her point, and the move is strengthened by the spontaneous flood of tears. This display could belong to any number of manipulative genteel women, who are ubiquitous in the Romantic-period novel, but precisely because of the text's sustained emphasis on Ethelinde's authentic sensibility, her behaviour tends to appear as sensitive and hurt feelings rather than as manipulation. This is confirmed by the way in which the chapter ends:

> Thus saying, Ethelinde arose, and still weeping excessively, left the room; whence Montgomery, who had already repented of having said what must give her pain, saw her depart without having courage to detain her, or attempt making his peace.[40]

Ethelinde's actions create a sense of acute distress, which adds force to her demand to relinquish the subject, making Montgomery regret his words, and perhaps causing him to doubt his own judgement because of the intensity of her denial. Because Ethelinde does, in fact, embody the theory of the elasticity of female nerves, it becomes impossible to separate the inherently exploitative nature of her actions from her hurt feelings. When Montgomery realizes he must have given Ethelinde pain he is entirely correct. Since she is Sir Edward's friend, Ethelinde's sensitive feelings are undoubtedly troubled by Montgomery's words. However, by this late in the story, it is clear that Ethelinde is fully conscious of Sir Edward's feelings for her, and her emotive denial of the situation is therefore a self-consciously manipulative attempt at maintaining the support necessary to her health. Ethelinde's sensitivity of feeling conceals the insensitivity of her actions.

The position of this exchange at the end of the chapter is provocative. Chapter endings in novels structure the story along lines of tempo and tone. The ending of the chapter creates a break in the storytelling, both because of the actual physical space at the end of the chapter which requires the reader to move to the next page to continue reading and because of the learnt assumption that a chapter ending signifies a break in content, tone or tempo, in much the same way as a paragraph break, only representing a more pronounced interruption. As a device which regulates tempo and tone, a chapter ending is primarily a feature of the telling of the story, and is therefore an aspect of the narrator's power. By ending the chapter with Ethelinde's dramatic exit, the narrator adds force to the heroine's emotive rhetoric, and places the reader in a similar position to Montgomery as Ethelinde makes her exit within the space of the text itself. Both reader and Montgomery are left with the image of the tearful and suffering Ethelinde as the last word of the chapter.

The next chapter, nevertheless, continues where the previous one ended, and mirrors it in tone:

> At the bottom of the stairs, where Ethelinde arrived almost without knowing where she went, or whither she intended to go, she met Miss Newenden. – 'Hey day!' cried the latter, 'what's the matter now? I never saw such a house in my life. There's Chesterville has been talking himself into a passion below, and you and Montgomery have been *sympathizing* above. It's altogether excessively wearing. Do have done with these perpetual lachrymals; really it hurts my spirits to hear of nothing but squabbling and sorrowing'.[41]

The reader is made to experience Ethelinde's distress more acutely because it punctuates the ending of the previous chapter, but by continuing the next chapter immediately where the previous one ended, the narrator maintains the picture of Ethelinde's suffering. The detailed, moment-by-moment, mimetic rendering of Ethelinde's actions and psychology does not allow the reader time to consider the detail of Montgomery's remarks in a way analogous to the analysis conducted above. Instead, the reader is encouraged to sympathize with Ethelinde as the narrator employs emotive rhetoric in concealing the truth of Montgomery's remarks in much the same way as Ethelinde does herself.

The chance meeting of Ethelinde with Miss Newenden (Nelly) is beyond the agency of both Ethelinde and narrator, being a fact of the story. On the one hand, Ethelinde's encounter with the symptomatically indelicate Nelly could serve to strengthen the reader's sympathy with Ethelinde. On the other, however, it is possible that Nelly actually clarifies the reader's growing disenchantment with the text's heroine and highlights the text's simultaneous embodiment and critique of the theory of sensibility. Throughout the text, Nelly operates as a plain-speaking voice which serves to undercut the plot of sensibility, such as in the passage cited. As a broadly sympathetic character, Nelly's negative comments on Ethelinde's actions cannot be as easily dismissed as those of the multiple vain and self-serving characters that populate the text. This is one of the first instances in the text in which the events of the story threaten to undermine Ethelinde's position. Reader perspective between the three levels of the reading experience becomes pertinent in producing the meaning of the text.

The dynamic between Ethelinde, Sir Edward and Lady Newenden is also implicated in the three reading levels of the text. The reader's understanding of this dynamic is complicated by the presentation of Mrs Montgomery's story, and the subplot of Nelly's marriage to Woolaston. Mrs Montgomery relates the story of her mother's lover, Lord Pevensey, who was not able to wed because he was already married to an insane woman (Lady Pevensey):

> 'to gratify his [Lord Pevensey's] family he had, when little more than twenty, married the heiress of a rich and noble family; plain, and even deformed in her person, with a temper soured by ill health and the consciousness of her own imperfections, and with manners the most disgusting. For upwards of three years he dragged on a life completely wretched with a woman whose malignity of temper deadened all pity for the personal misfortune. At the end of that period she was seized with the small pox, attended with the worst symptoms: but the distemper acting on a habit perpetually bad, failed to deprive her of life, which would have been a blessing to them both; but left behind it violent epileptic fits, which ... deprived her of the slender share of reason she ever possessed, and threw her at length into confirmed idiotism'.[42]

The text draws an explicit link between physical health and the mind. Lady Pevensey's 'temper is soured by ill health', and she survives smallpox because of her perpetually bad habits. In contradistinction to Colonel Chesterville, who experiences increased melancholic sympathy for those around him because of his desperate financial situation, and who quietly accepts his fate well before his illness claims his life, Lady Pevensey rather experiences an increased hardness of heart which in some degree protects her from smallpox. The associations with sensibility are strong, with the text implying that such tough nerves only lead to a poisoned mind and resilience to illness which is paradoxically seen as a curse (after all, it would have been a blessing if Lady Pevensey had died). This formulation of hard nerves as undesirable, and of sensibility as grace, is once again undercut, however. On the one hand, Lady Pevensey is presented in such negative terms that the reader is invited to overlook the fact that Lord Pevensey and Mrs Montgomery's mother are not married and thus are living in sin. On the other hand, the very dark imagery employed to describe the abject condition of the discarded Lady Pevensey, left as she is disfigured and suffering fits alone in an insane asylum, disrupts the reader's sense of the propriety of the actions of Lord Pevensey and his lover. There is an obvious similarity in this story with that of Sir Edward, Ethelinde and Lady Newenden. Lady Newenden is also a wife eclipsed by a love rival, she is also presented very negatively, and her ending is no doubt a tragic one: she ultimately dies a 'sudden death'.[43]

Lady Newenden's marriage to Sir Edward rescues him financially. Similarly, Lady Pevensey is rich, and it is implied that this is a primary reason why Lord Pevensey's family urged the alliance. Nelly also brings money to her marriage, restoring Woolaston's wealth. All three women end tragically (as well as the sorry ends of Lady Newenden and Lady Pevensey described above, Nelly is swindled of her fortune and subject to domestic violence). In terms of the plot, the stories of Lady Pevensey's and Nelly's marriages resonate with and add nuance to the reader's understanding of the primary love triangle between Ethelinde, Sir Edward and Lady Newenden. The dark imagery in Mrs Montgomery's backstory (which is crucially reported by Mrs Montgomery, not the narrator, thus sidestepping the narrator's power to influence the reader in favour of Ethelinde), and the tragic ends of the three women described, disrupt the narrator's endorsement of the relationship between Sir Edward and Ethelinde, implicitly questioning the desirability of Ethelinde's sensibility.

One of the main challenges Ethelinde faces in forging a future life is in balancing her romantic desire for Montgomery with her need for Sir Edward's financial and social support. The nuances of narrative control that this predicament engenders are perhaps most clear in an episode concerning a miniature painting of Ethelinde, which both men want to own. Montgomery asks Ethelinde for the picture to take with him when he goes abroad to seek his fortune:

> A blush rose on the check of Ethelinde; and faltering she said – 'Indeed, Montgomery, I would give you the picture with pleasure – but I have not got it'.
>
> 'Who has it then?' said he eagerly. 'Have you given it to Chesterville?'
>
> 'No', replied Ethelinde, who by this question had an opportunity of concealing the truth, had she been capable of artifice, 'but Sir Edward, who is fond of Meyer's miniatures, and thought that, not only very like but extremely well painted, begged me to have it'.[44]

There is reason to mistrust the narrator's insistence on Ethelinde's integrity here, since it is unlikely that she exactly tells the truth concerning Sir Edward's motives for wanting the miniature, as suggested by her blushing and faltering speech. By this late point in the story, it is absolutely certain that Ethelinde fully understands Sir Edward's feelings towards her, meaning she would know that he wanted the miniature because it was of her rather than because of its artistic merit. It is possible, and probably factual, that Sir Edward had given Ethelinde the reasons for wanting the picture that she then reports to Montgomery, since to openly avow his love would not only be futile but also likely result in his permanent separation from Ethelinde. For her part, Ethelinde knows this, and knows therefore that she is in no danger of losing Sir Edward's support so long as he feels for her as he does but does not make his feelings explicit. This assertion is borne out by Ethelinde's numerous attempts to maintain Sir Edward's marriage with Lady Newenden, since the failure of the marriage would put her in danger of a receiving a proposal from Sir Edward. The miniature would typically be stored in a locket worn around the neck, and even though Sir Edward does not wear it but 'has merely put it into a little cabinet where he keeps many others'[45] (or at least this is what he claims), the romantic associations are strong. Even so, since Sir Edward probably only gives artistic reasons for wanting to possess the miniature (since, as stated, anything more romantically explicit would effectively force Ethelinde to relinquish his gifts, which neither wish for), Ethelinde has not said anything that did not happen in reality, and is able to diminish the gift's romantic connotations.

It is also notable that Ethelinde's gift of the picture to Sir Edward occurs offstage. The giving of the picture is a fact of the story, but the decision to represent it behind the scenes belongs to the narrator. In the overall context of the different levels of reader perception regarding Ethelinde, this move is highly suggestive. Given the narrator's consistent support of the heroine, it is possible to imagine a more coquettish Ethelinde than the narrator would care to have us see in the act of giving the picture, and perhaps a more overtly romantic Sir Edward, than is seen in the mimetically represented action of *Ethelinde*. The narrator's decision to brush over the event suggests a wish to draw a veil over this aspect of story. The effect is heightened by the fact that this is the only place in the entire story in which the narrator alludes to a scene between Ethelinde and Sir Edward occurring offstage, suggestive of a world of secret correspondence occurring outside of the reported story. In fact, it would seem that since the picture episode implicates several characters, its description cannot be avoided by the narrator without leaving holes in the plot. The events of the story have conspired against both Ethelinde and the narrator and offer the reader a perspective outside of their combined influence.

If the above considerations cast doubt over Ethelinde's sincerity, then the following explicitly contradicts the narrator's claim that she is incapable 'of artifice':[46]

> after much deliberation [Ethelinde] determined to ask Sir Edward for [the miniature] the next morning, that she might leave it in town to be copied ... she fixed on this plan; and she knew [Montgomery] had never seen the picture above twice, and that she could have it very exactly copied, she believed he would not distinguish it from the original; and should by this means gratify Montgomery without appearing capricious and ungrateful to Sir Edward Newenden.[47]

Possibly the clearest presentation of Ethelinde's self-interested behaviour in the text, here the narrator is forced to acknowledge that Ethelinde self-consciously manages the competing claims of Montgomery and Sir Edward so as to maintain both her romantic interest in Montgomery and the financial support of Sir Edward, both of which are pertinent to her future health. The unexpected request from Montgomery for the miniature upsets Ethelinde's position and plan. She is forced into insincerity and subterfuge to maintain the interests essential to her emotional and financial health. This in turn places the narrator in an equally uncomfortable position; he/she can find no spin to mystify Ethelinde's manipulation. All that can do done is to insist that Ethelinde is incapable of artifice because she does not allow Montgomery to assume that her brother, Chesterville, possesses the miniature when given the chance, but the narrator is still forced to describe Ethelinde's plan of intrigue because of its pertinence to the plot of the story.

The narrator, nevertheless, is able to moderate Ethelinde's indiscretion by drawing attention to Montgomery's conduct. Ethelinde successfully convinces Montgomery that his jealousy of Sir Edward has been untoward, 'but the picture, the picture, like the handkerchief of Othello, was still not to be got over'.[48] The 'weeping and distressed Ethelinde was at length compelled to promise that she would ask Sir Edward for it',[49] and yet Montgomery 'made her again and again repeat the promise'.[50] Montgomery's whining desperation is emphasized by the repetition of the phrase 'the picture, the picture', conveying a tone of self-pitying despondency. The allusion to *Othello*, which relates to an instance of romantic jealousy 'that soon turns into murderous rage',[51] gives Montgomery's envy a hyperbolic quality, casting it as immature. Ethelinde appears to be forced into a concession arising from pity for a distressed boy. This effect is primarily caused by the narrator, who creates the tone of the passage by the language employed.

Sir Edward forces Ethelinde into a similar position. Ethelinde explains she wishes to have a copy made of the miniature for Montgomery:

> Sir Edward changed countenance; but said, as calmly as he could – 'I will fetch the picture, Ethelinde; perhaps you may chuse to give Mr. Montgomery that rather than a copy. If so, I am sure *my* wish to keep it ought to yield to his and yours'.
>
> He suppressed a sigh, and arose. Ethelinde, who could not bear to see him unhappy, answered – 'No, Sir Edward, if it is of the least value to you as a good miniature I would by no means take it'. She was confused, and hardly knew what she ought to say ...
>
> Sir Edward felt that it were wiser not to retain it; but he could not prevail on himself to resign it to Montgomery.[52]

From a purely moral standpoint, it is Ethelinde who should take a stand here. Sir Edward is willing to give up the picture should she desire it, and it is probably harder for him to press the decision on Ethelinde than it is for her to demand it, if only because of the unrequited love on his side. This would serve to make clearer to all parties the distinction between Montgomery as lover and Sir Edward as guardian and friend. However, it is essential that Sir Edward's romantic feelings remain strong if Ethelinde is to continue to exploit the financial and social assets from him which remain essential to her health, and as such Ethelinde wants Sir Edward to keep the picture. Moreover, if Sir Edward were to find the strength to cut his ties with Ethelinde then she would likely be the target of gossip, since Sir Edward's sudden rupture with Ethelinde would (correctly) appear as a direct result of the unrequited love on his side, potentially causing acute emotional stress which, as we have seen, may mean serious physical illness for the those with high levels of sensibility. Despite the inherent self-interest in Ethelinde's actions, however, her evident desire to mitigate Sir Edward's hurt in the passage cited works to erase the sense of her self-interest, as does the narrator's explicit statement that Ethelinde could not bear to see Sir Edward unhappy.

The reader is reminded of the miniature once more just over a hundred pages later. This is part of Montgomery's account of his arduous journey from the East Indies back to England:

> 'and at night, or whenever my watch was over, I kissed the two dear pictures I had preserved of my mother and my Ethelinde: their beloved images soothed my short slumbers, and I awoke indeed to new toils, but to toil lightened by the hope of soon embracing the beloved originals'.[53]

Montgomery's comfort in his picture is founded on a lie, and the reader is reminded of this by his reference to the 'originals', which acquires significance for the reader if it is remembered that this picture is in fact a copy of a copy, and that Sir Edward has the first copy. Notably the narrator attempts to protect Ethelinde by refusing to remind the reader of the picture's import, but has no power to alter Montgomery's unfortunate (from the narrator's perspective) choice of words, which are a fact of the story.

This chapter has demonstrated how the eighteenth-century theory of sensibility is powerfully implicated in questions of health in *Ethelinde*. Moreover, the text implicitly critiques the equation of sensibility with altruism. Genuine sensibility – and the capacity to empathize with others it potentially generates – can be used in the service of self rather than others; paradoxically, the very empathy which defines it is implicated in unfeeling behaviour exerted for self-gain. In *Ethelinde*, this exploitation of the sensibility of the nerves is always related to health. Those with great sensibility are in great danger from emotional and physical distress, and yet it is precisely Ethelinde's exploitation of her sensibility which allows her to avoid the financial destitution which ultimately kills her father: sensibility turns out to be both the cause and preventative medication of illness.

This presentation of health is pictured through a challenging narrative technique that situates the reader between competing levels of the reading experience. Ethelinde's self-interested behaviour is mystified in the act of telling as the narrator presents the reader with a specific view of Ethelinde's actions, in the effects of random events external to Ethelinde's own agency, and under the cultural resonance of her own putative embodiment of Romantic-period sensibility and the associations of feeling for others it encodes. *Ethelinde* implicitly critiques the theory of sensibility by revealing the possible ways behaviour within its framework is subject to radically different interpretations. Ultimately, the text makes no judgement on Ethelinde's actions. Its competing levels of representation do not allow for an authoritative moral standpoint. Rather, readers are asked to picture Ethelinde's struggle for health and formulate judgements for themselves. This value judgement asks questions of the reader's own ideological standpoint. As a genteel lady culturally excluded from wage-labour, Ethelinde's actions may be the only way she can achieve not only her personal goals, but also ensure her continued good health, implicitly questioning the class and gender formations in the period which exclude her from paid labour, and the amalgamation of capitalist and feudal modes of production which permit self-interested behaviour in the productive sphere but which condemn it within polite, leisured society. For all that, there is no doubt that Ethelinde exploits others to achieve her goals, and most readers, I would contend, would find her actions at least a little distasteful if not outright immoral. *Ethelinde*, then, is a novel that implicates questions of health in serious moral judgements on the part of reader.

2 AMAZONIAN FASHIONS: LADY DELACOUR'S (RE)DRESS IN MARIA EDGEWORTH'S *BELINDA*[1]

Andrew McInnes

In the course of Edgeworth's 1801 novel *Belinda*, the fashionable Lady Delacour suffers from sexual, physical and mental health problems caused, in part, by her dissipated London lifestyle. First, she becomes entangled in the pseudo-feminist Harriet Freke's homoerotic desires and cross-dressing; political campaigns; and a duel with her female rival, Mrs Luttridge, which results in a self-inflicted wound to her breast. Because she disguises this wound and consults a trendy quack doctor, Lady Delacour's health declines throughout the novel almost to the point of death. Poorly prepared for her seemingly imminent demise, Lady Delacour turns in desperation to Methodism, which causes delusions exploited by her one-time friend, Freke.

The original plan of Edgeworth's novel climaxes in Lady Delacour's tragic death, providing a somewhat clichéd conclusion to a standard anti-fashion satire. Her survival, rehabilitation and, indeed, triumph in the published novel cause havoc with Edgeworth's moralistic framework. Lady Delacour's redress hinges on her own overt questioning of the healthiness of the female body, the naturalness of her position as wife and mother, and, in a startlingly metatextual manoeuvre, the marriage plot of the eighteenth-century novel itself, revealing each to be fashionable constructs. Lady Delacour orchestrates the final scene of the novel, challenging both characters and readers with her final words, 'Our *tale* contains a *moral*, and no doubt, / You all have wit enough to find it out'.[2] I argue that Lady Delacour's witty questioning of morals and manners in contemporary tales reveals both to depend upon the fashionable ideologies underpinning modern society, from the medical imperative for mothers to breastfeed their children, to men's desire for a 'natural' woman untainted by 'fashion', to the mechanics of the eighteenth-century marriage plot itself.

In this chapter, I analyse Edgeworth's picturing of women's health in relation to the picturing of women in visual culture, particularly in James Gillray's satires of fashion, which often focus unhealthily on women's breasts; contemporary medical discourse on women's health, especially debates about breastfeeding which become contentiously intertwined to responses to the French Revolution throughout the 1790s; and religious polemic which sought to connect Methodism to mental illness in the same period. The seemingly disparate realms of graphic satires, medical treatises and religious polemics testify to the extent to which contemporary anxieties about the healthiness of women's bodies penetrated popular consciousness in the period. In *Belinda*, Edgeworth draws on these popular conceptions of the female form to represent Lady Delacour's (un)healthy body as a matrix including expressions of sexual desire; physical strength and integrity; emotional receptivity; and spiritual and mental resolve. These aspects of her health are tested to the point of destruction by the wound to her breast. For Edgeworth, then, a women's breast forms a locus around which these sexual, physical, emotional and spiritual health issues are particularly fraught, open to contestation, especially repressive social constructions which seek to limit women's agency. The breast is at once a sexual object; an indicator of maternity and maternal sentiment; and can be accentuated or disguised by women's fashions. Lady Delacour's overt questioning of social conventions surrounding the supposed naturalness of women's bodies accesses fashionable language to reveal the artifice behind assertions of female 'nature' which seek to render women passive, obedient, sexualized subjects.

Maria Edgeworth (1768–1849) was a prolific Anglo-Irish novelist, who also published poetry, short stories, children's fiction and educational treatises, sometimes in collaboration with her polymath father Richard Lovell Edgeworth (1744–1817). She was one of the most popular writers of the early nineteenth century, her work easily eclipsing both the sales and critical reception of the lesser-known Jane Austen and inspiring the historical fiction of Walter Scott. Like Jane Austen, she has been categorized as a conservative, if not simply Anti-Jacobin, writer, most influentially by Marilyn Butler, although twenty-first-century criticism, especially Cliona Ó Gallchoir's definitive critical biography, has repositioned her as more liberal, challenging and subversive.[3] James Gillray (1757–1815) was a prolific printmaker, producing hundreds, if not thousands, of violently imaginative, phantasmagoric caricatures of politicians; celebrities; current events, especially the bloody excesses of the French Revolution; and fashionable London life. Throughout the 1780s and into the early 1790s he produced several graphic satires caricaturing the actress, poet, novelist and radical writer, Mary Robinson (1757–1800), positioning her in an increasingly sexualized manner next to political and society figures, including her lover, the future George IV; James Cecil, the Lord Chamberlain; and his wife, Mary Amelia Cecil in 'Monuments Lately Discovered on Salisbury Plain' (1782); George again and the opposition politician Charles James Fox in 'Paridise [*sic*] Regain'd' (1783); and her lover Banastre Tarleton and George yet again in 'The Thunderer' (1792). In this last print, Robinson is displayed, legs splayed, as a 'whirligig' shop-sign, crudely representing her sexual availability. Gillray's misogynistic images of her played their part in the picturing of the sexual and physical health of her body. Robinson took an active role engaging with representations of herself in pop culture, reclaiming her body from polyvocal perspectives in poetry, prose and polemic. Like Mary Robinson, Lady Delacour is a lady of fashion, represented by herself and others as a sexually desirable object. Like Robinson, Edgeworth's lady of fashion strives to reclaim her body from cultural constructions of femininity, maternity and fashionable life.

Edgeworth herself occupies an ambiguous position in relation to 1790s culture and politics, similar to Robinson's caricaturist, Gillray. From the late 1790s onwards, Gillray's visual satires were secretly sponsored by the British government. In light of this, he has been read as a profoundly conservative artist, supporting the Pitt government's oppressive response to the French revolutionary threat, although Gillray's art approaches at its best a carnivalesque anarchy, at worst despairing nihilism, continuing as he does to viciously satirize his paymasters. Indeed, Mark Hallett argues that

> [t]his alliance between Gillray's satire and the purposes of journalistic propaganda has often been dismissed as a regrettable and diminished phase of his life and career. On the contrary, it generated some of Gillray's most artistically brilliant and inventive images.[4]

Summing up the difficulties Victorian and more modern critics have had evaluating both Gillray's oeuvre and his oscillating reputation, Diana Donald posits this fascinating image:

> Gillray the inspired genius, Gillray the unprincipled hireling – like one of those puzzle drawings in which two different images are separately perceptible, but impossible to hold in the mind simultaneously, his caricatures caused, and still cause, an acute apprehension of disturbance and conflict.[5]

Juxtaposing Edgeworth's sophisticated fiction with Gillray's grotesque satires, especially his images of women and fashion in the period, reveals a surprising overlap in style: both Edgeworth and Gillray present seemingly conservative images of women and dress, whilst their work contains more challenging and subversive energies.

Critical engagement with *Belinda* focuses on Edgeworth's treatments of fashion and domesticity, nature and artifice, morality and satire in the novel, with interpretations often hinging either explicitly or implicitly on picturing the health of Lady Delacour's breast. Readings of the novel as a conservative moral tale focus on Lady Delacour's wounded breast as symbolic of her punishment as a fashionable lady neglecting her position as wife and mother, and her (and her breast's) recovery as reinscribing her into domestic discourse. For example, Susan Greenfield argues that

> when Lady Delacour finally allows her body to be circulated among men, the revelation that her breast is normal beneath the surface injury, that the organ is internally pure, rectifies the system of sexual difference the wound had challenged and proves that unfeminine behaviour cannot change a woman's essence.[6]

Through rereading Edgeworth's treatment of fashion and artifice, I seek to challenge Greenfield's contention that the movement of *Belinda* is to reify 'a woman's essence'. I am more sympathetic to analyses of Lady Delacour which seek to account for the more subversive energies in the novel: these readings explore the fashionable woman's resistance to male-dominated medical discourse and Lady Delacour's subsequent suspicion of the conventional morality subordinating women to a passive role in the private sphere. For example, Ruth Perry argues against earlier readings of Lady Delacour's wounded breast as betraying 'guilt over her failure to nurse her child' by suggesting that it 'could also be read as festering resentment at the colonization of her body'.[7] Indeed, what unites both Kelly and Greenfield's divergent readings is a focus on the colonial implications of Lady Delacour's physical health and social position.

Lady Delacour's wounded breast and the way in which it is healed form the crux, depending on whether one reads the wound or its healing as implicating Lady Delacour in the colonization of women's bodies, of a series of postcolonial readings of Edgeworth's novel, linking her critique of the hypocritical standards of female propriety with colonial anxieties about race, miscegenation and imperial rule explored in *Belinda*. Along with Susan Greenfield, Andrew McCann and Kathryn Kirkpatrick both add to the debate about the significance of Edgeworth's colonial concerns to her feminist arguments in *Belinda*. McCann complicates Greenfield's argument that Lady Delacour, reinscribed at the novel's conclusion as a 'proper lady', acts as guarantor of colonial advantage and gender difference.[8] By focusing on the differences between 1801 and 1810 editions of the novel, McCann argues that the earlier edition questioned both colonial advantage and gender difference, especially in the positive representation of the marriage between Mr Vincent's black slave Juba and a working-class white woman, which Edgeworth hints is a progressive, healthy development for English class-bound, exclusive society.[9] My focus on Lady Delacour's criticisms of the fashionable world and fashionable models of domesticity brings McCann's postcolonial focus closer to home. Kirkpatrick analyses the reasons behind Edgeworth's revisions, focusing on the equivocation of Edgeworth's explanation for removing Juba's marriage from the text: 'My father says that gentlemen have horrors upon this subject, and would draw conclusions very unfavourable to a female writer who appeared to recommend such unions: as I do not understand the subject I trust to his better judgement'. Kirkpatrick argues that Edgeworth has shown a very precise understanding of the conflation of sexual and racial anxieties in her novel. Therefore, her lack of understanding focuses on the personal horrors of the gentlemen rather than any horror she feels towards the subject of interracial marriage.[10] I build on Kirkpatrick's sense of Edgeworth's sophistication as a novelist to argue that she creates, in Lady Delacour, a character almost metatextually aware of her status as a fiction, manipulating a conventional marriage plot for her own ends. I have a different focus from McCann and Kirkpatrick, but engage with their rereadings of *Belinda* in order to argue, contra Greenfield, that Lady Delacour distinguishes herself from the 'proper lady' by persistently questioning categorizations of acceptable behaviour for women, especially wives and mothers, revealing them to depend on fashionable constructs.

I find Cliona Ó Gallchoir's characterization of the novel as having 'the quality of a kaleidoscope, in which flashing images of belles, beaux, rakes, fops, servants, conjurers, colonials and émigrés pass before our eyes in sometimes bewildering sequence' useful in broadening the scope of *Belinda* beyond the pedestrian travails of its protagonist to the kaleidoscopic perspectives on contemporary femininity embodied by Harriet Freke, Lady Delacour and Virginia de St Pierre, especially Edgeworth's representation of the fashionable world, within which Lady Delacour takes an increasingly controlling position both of the beau monde and the novel itself.[11] Further, Susan Egenolf reads this metatextuality as indicative of Edgeworth's personal involvement in politically charged polemic, arguing that the artistic glosses in the novel reveal political manoeuvres by which women can maintain control over their lives.[12] I argue that Lady Delacour maintains her controlling position within the text, both as an influential, fashionable figure in high society and as a character who increasingly takes an orchestrating role in the novel's climax and denouement, by triumphing over the sexual, physical and mental health issues which beset her at the novel's beginning, in her assertion of control over the healthiness of her own body.

Gillray's print 'The Fashionable Mamma; or, The Convenience of Modern Dress' published in the same year as 'Lady Godina's Rout' echoes several themes in *Belinda*, especially the question of balancing the requirements of fashionable society with the demands and responsibilities of being a mother. Gillray's depiction of a fashionably dressed woman passively allowing her child to breastfeed through slits in her dress, whilst a maid does the work of supporting the infant, once more seems to comment censoriously on the flimsiness of modern fashions and a matching lassitude in women's moral fibre, whilst asking its audience to gaze, with the gentleman caller peering through the window, on the woman's exposed breasts. Edgeworth's novel has nothing close to such an explicit and overtly titillating scene, with the revelation of Lady Delacour's breast described only as a 'hideous spectacle' rather than pornographically visualized as in Gillray's print.[13] The connection between Edgeworth's novel and Gillray's print resides in their joint awareness of the absurdity of the link made between women's fashions and their responsibilities as mothers, with the sexualized nature of Gillray's fashionable mamma contrasting with and impeding her expected role in caring for her child. Edgeworth takes this absurdity a step further than Gillray by suggesting that the imposition of maternal breastfeeding by medical practitioners is itself only a fashion.

Ruth Perry's excellent article 'Colonizing the Breast: Sexuality and Maternity in Eighteenth-Century England' offers a comprehensive account of the way '[t]he medical focus on maternal breastfeeding [in the period] can be interpreted as the beginning of the physiological colonization of women's bodies corresponding to the psychological colonization of women's subjectivity in both companionate marriage and motherhood',[14] concluding with a reading of Edgeworth's novel, especially Lady Delacour's wounded breast, as offering resistance to this model. Building on Perry's thesis, I want to reread several key moments she identifies in eighteenth-century thinking about women's breasts as the site of a conflict between nature and artifice, or fashion. Perry reads a series of texts advocating breastfeeding in which a mother breastfeeding her own child is read as natural, whilst the practice of hiring a wet nurse is considered a fashionable flaw, linked to a vain attempt to maintain a false standard of female beauty. For example, she quotes William Cadogan's influential *An Essay upon Nursing, and the Management of Children, From Their Birth to Three Years* (1748) as urging every woman to 'prevail upon herself to give up a little of the Beauty of her Breast to feed her Offspring'.[15] Later, in 1784, Michael Underwood, a fashionable man-midwife to several prominent women of the day, including Caroline of Brunswick, argues in *A Treatise on the Diseases of Children* that '[t]hat tyrant, Fashion [for wet nursing] has prevailed over the good sense and natural feelings of many whose maternal affections can be in no other instance, suspected'.[16] Mary Wollstonecraft in her 1792 *A Vindication of the Rights of Woman* argues that women avoid breastfeeding '[t]o preserve their beauty, and wear the flowery crown of the day'.[17] Edgeworth's focus on nature and fashion throughout *Belinda* leads her to the more sophisticated point that the polemical focus on maternal breastfeeding is as much a fashionable construct as the earlier convention of wet-nursing. *Belinda* consistently questions what it means to be 'natural', with Lady Delacour as the novel's most vocal proponent of the societal, fashionable construction of a woman's nature, in particular.

Throughout the novel, Lady Delacour comments acerbically on her lack of success as a mother whilst she attempts to maintain her position in fashionable society. This criticism is directed both at her own perceived failings as a woman and on the social codes which demand that women be both caring mothers and leading members of society – these dictates lead to her declining physical, emotional and mental health. Lady Delacour's anxieties about breastfeeding predate the wound to her breast which motivates the rest of her narrative. Before explaining the series of events which lead up to this wound, she relates to Belinda the tragic history of her first two children, a boy who was stillborn and the second a girl, described as 'but a poor, diminutive, sickly thing'.[18] Lady Delacour suggestively connects the healthiness of this female child with the debates surrounding the extent to which breastfeeding was natural or fashionable for eighteenth-century mothers:

> It was the fashion at this time for fine mothers to suckle their own children – so much the worse for the poor brats ... There was a prodigious rout made about the matter; a vast deal of sentiment and sympathy, and compliments and inquiries; but after the novelty was over, I became heartily sick of the business; and at the end of about three months my poor child was sick too – I don't much like to think of it – it died. If I had put it out to nurse, I should have been thought an unnatural mother – but I should have saved its life.[19]

Lady Delacour makes it clear in her narration that she followed the fashion for maternal breastfeeding against her better judgement, under threat of being thought an 'unnatural mother'. Maternal breastfeeding is surrounded by fashionable terminology in this passage, described as a 'novelty' producing a 'prodigious rout' and creating a buzz of sentiment and compliments. The result of following the fashion in medical discourse here leads to the death of her daughter, whereas Lady Delacour states that the frowned-upon, unfashionable wet-nursing would have saved her.

In recounting the rest of her history to Belinda, Lady Delacour pinpoints the origin of the health issues which beset her throughout the novel as her implicitly sexual attraction to Harriet Freke, presented as a seductively transvestite feminist. Freke's influence on Lady Delacour's behaviour is accounted for as a combination of domestic neglect, fashionable manners and erotic frisson. Lady Delacour specifies that she 'has nothing at home, either in the shape of husband or children, to engage my affections'.[20] In his chapter in this collection, Joseph Morrissey argues that Smith's eponymous heroine challenges contemporary codes of feminine propriety through her extreme conformity to them; I argue that Lady Delacour subverts them by revealing their artificial, constructed, fashionable character. Both Smith and Edgeworth represent these codes of feminine behaviour as damaging to a woman's health, with Smith showing how Ethelinde has to find ways around them through manipulation and Edgeworth deconstructing the societal hypocrisy which puts pressure on women's sexual, emotional, physical and spiritual health.

Indeed, Lady Delacour's emphasis on domesticity when she laments her empty home life only seems to shore up readings of *Belinda* as moralizingly conservative,

Lady Delacour's stipulation that she believed 'it was this "aching void" in my heart which made me... take such a prodigious fancy to Mrs Freke' positions the absence of domestic affections in ironic, distancing scare quotes. She continues:

> [Harriet Freke] was just then coming into fashion – she struck me the first time I met her, as being downright ugly; but there was a wild oddity in her countenance which made one stare at her, and she was delighted to be stared at – especially by me – so we were mutually agreeable to each other – I as starer, and she as staree. Harriet Freke had, without comparison, more assurance than any man or woman I ever saw ... She was one of the first who brought what I call *harum scarum* manners into fashion.[21]

Again, Lady Delacour's focus on Freke's fashionability seems to fit readings of *Belinda* as an anti-fashion satire: Lady Delacour's homoerotic attraction towards Freke – implicit in Freke's delight in being stared at by her and their mutual agreeableness – leads to Lady Delacour's dangerous flirtation with another man (who is then killed in a duel with Lord Delacour) and her own duel with Mrs Luttridge, which climaxes in her self-inflicted wound to her breast. Indeed, Lisa Moore argues that Edgeworth is both conservative and homophobic in her aggressive containment of Freke's expressions of lesbian desire in the novel, climaxing in her disfigurement in a mantrap leading to the end of her cross-dressing.[22] However, Lady Delacour's representation of her intense female friendship with Freke moves beyond a simplistic and reductive depiction of sexual perversion leading to physical and emotional health problems, and forms part of her questioning of the social construction of femininity. Whilst Freke's explicit homoeroticism is violently policed within the novel, Lady Delacour's implicit bisexuality remains permissible and subversive. Moreover, her focus on manners, explicitly linked to fashion and artifice throughout the novel, here chimes with her earlier dismissal of morals, implicitly connected to social constructions of 'healthy' femininity, which will be echoed in the novel's own conclusion. She begins her story with the moral 'a woman who is known to play the fool, is always suspected of playing the devil', continuing

> But I begin where I ought to end, with my moral, which I dare say you are not impatient to anticipate – I never read or listened to a moral at the end of a story in my life – manners for me, and morals for those who like them.[23]

By continually stressing manners over morals, Lady Delacour aligns herself with fashion against domesticity. Fashion is problematic and troubling in *Belinda*, but then, so is domesticity, and Lady Delacour constantly shows how the two terms are inextricably interlinked, revealing late eighteenth-century ideals of domesticity to be fashionable constructs. Throughout the novel, Lady Delacour proves herself to be a shrewd reader of manners and morals, fashion and domesticity, showing that her engagement with the fashionable world has not blinded her to either Freke's or her own flaws.

Immediately after Lady Delacour critiques morals and manners, she disavows her life's resemblance to fiction: 'My dear, you will be woefully disappointed, if in my story you expect any thing like a novel'.[24] However, she is aware that her history, sometimes painfully, resembles a play. Recounting the circumstances of her duel with Mrs Luttridge, Lady Delacour exclaims:

> Life is a tragicomedy! Though the critics will allow of no such thing in their books, it is a true representation of what passes in the world; and of all lives, mine has been the most grotesque mixture, or alternation, I should say, of tragedy and comedy ... This comic duel ended tragically for me ... I was not used to priming and loading – my pistol was overcharged – when I fired it recoiled, and I received a blow on my breast, the consequences of which you have seen – or are to see.[25]

Lady Delacour maintains a sophisticated sense of the performative nature of her actions, linking her self-inflicted wound to the breast to the mixed genre of tragicomedy. By staging her own life in this way, she seeks to maintain control both of her own actions and the behaviour and opinions of the other characters in the novel, taking an increasingly directorial role in Edgeworth's plot as it progresses. Edgeworth's engagement with the theatre throughout her works has been read together with her statements on fashion as placing her within the tradition of conservative satire.[26] However, more recent work has complicated Edgeworth's position by pointing out that themes of play-acting, performance and theatricality are treated more sympathetically and rigorously than this allows. For example, Terry Robinson offers a more sophisticated approach to the novel in '"Life is a Tragicomedy!": Maria Edgeworth's *Belinda* and the Staging of the Realist Novel', reading its engagement with the theatre, in terms of dramatic practice and stage management, as paradoxically guaranteeing the realist novel's authenticity effect.[27] Although I agree with Robinson that Edgeworth's treatment of the theatre is much more sympathetic than has been previously allowed, my focus is on the very inauthenticity such effects give to the novel and the fashionable constructs within it. Throughout the novel, Lady Delacour maintains her actorly persona, even taking on a directorial role towards the denouement. Edgeworth's more complex use of the theatre, alongside her developing interest in fashion, makes for a more subversive reading of *Belinda*, one which, instead of condemning theatricality and performance, foregrounds the extent to which even seemingly 'natural' aspects of femininity, conventionally represented as healthy, depend on artifice, considered unhealthy in traditional anti-theatre polemic. Lady Delacour's focus on fashion, artifice and performance seeks to free her body from social conventions seeking to dictate 'natural', 'healthy' behaviour, instead asserting performative control over her own actions.

The immediate consequences of Lady Delacour's tragicomic duel with Mrs Luttridge is that both women are attacked by a mob enraged less by the fact of a female duel than by their apparel whilst fighting it. Lady Delacour is scathing in her treatment of the lower-class crowd, stating that they were 'so shocked at the idea of a duel fought by women in *men's clothes*' and condemning them as 'Stupid blockheads! I am convinced that they would not have been half so much scandalized if we had boxed in our petticoats'.[28] Lady Delacour's fashionable status, informing both her snobbery and sophisticated dress sense here, enables her to give telling insights into how gender is constructed through clothes, demonstrating that conventional morality pays as much attention to clothing as those more interested in manners and societal codes of behaviour.

Lady Delacour concludes her tragicomic life story by admitting the decline in her health and the demise of her friendship with Harriet Freke. Belinda notices that her friend seems to be in great pain. Lady Delacour responds:

> O! – I am, sometimes ... as you see, in terrible pain. For two years after I gave myself that blow with the pistol, I neglected the warning twinges that I felt from time to time – at last I was terrified.[29]

Refusing to consult a physician, she decides on a course of dissipation to avoid acrimonious reflections, stating ruefully: 'Conscience! conscience will be heard. Since my health has been weakened, I believe I have acquired more conscience'.[30] This realization also leads to a break with Freke, who betrays her trust to associate with Mrs Luttridge. Lady Delacour tells Belinda that her former friend 'has cost me my peace of mind – my health – my life'.[31] It is the loss of this peace of mind which has the most significant impact on her health and life, as Lady Delacour's mental disequilibrium leads her towards religious enthusiasm and the brink of death.

Later in the novel, Belinda catches Lady Delacour reading John Wesley's *Admonitions*, one of the Methodist minister's many publications. The fourth Admonition, 'Advice to an Unhappy Woman', exactly echoes Lady Delacour's anxieties about the state of her physical and spiritual health at that point in the novel. Wesley begins with a series of questions: 'Whither are you going? To heaven or hell? Do you not know? Do you never think about it? Why do you not? Are you never to die? Nay, it is appointed for all men to die'. Throughout the short piece, Wesley focuses on women's bodies: 'Know ye not, that your body is, or ought to be, the temple of the Holy Ghost which is in you?', stressing that a dissipated lifestyle leads to 'Destruction both of body and soul'.[32] Wesley's Methodist imprecations to women to consider the healthiness of their bodies and souls provide another way of picturing the significance of women's health, particularly that of fashionable ladies like Delacour, in the period.

Edgeworth presents Lady Delacour's entanglement with Methodism as the most serious test of her healthy mind and body:

> During the solitude of her illness, her ladyship had first begun to think seriously on religious subjects, and the early impressions that had been made on her mind in her childhood, by a methodistical mother, recurred. Her understanding, weakened perhaps by disease, and never accustomed to reason, was incapable of distinguishing between truth and errour [*sic*]; and her temper, naturally enthusiastic, hurried her from one extreme to the other – from thoughtless scepticism to visionary credulity.[33]

Edgeworth specifies here that Lady Delacour is drawn to the faith through memories of a 'methodistical mother', perhaps an oblique way of shoring up Lady Delacour's own earlier criticisms of the suitability of upper-class women to nurse their own children. In any case, Lady Delacour's fashionable flirtation with Methodism threatens her mental health, already weakened by physical illness. As the wound to her breast will soon be revealed as not as serious as she feared, it becomes Lady Delacour's irrational dependence on religious enthusiasm which is truly dangerous to both her health and the fragile equilibrium of her private life. Anxieties surrounding the growing popularity of, or fashion for, Methodism, a liberal creed actively welcoming women as preachers, were prevalent in the late eighteenth century, with several eminent writers and clerics warning against the fragmentation in faith the movement seemed to herald. To explain these fears surrounding Methodism, Richard Polwhele's *Anecdotes of Methodism* provides an insight into the range of concerns circulating about this fast-developing faith in the late eighteenth century. Writing as a Church of England minister of a Cornish town, his 'eye-witness' account of Cornishmen and women turning to the new religion concludes by categorizing a number of revealing side effects of Methodism, including:

> Ignorance with itching ears, Prevarication, Lying, Hypocrisy, Knavery, Contempt of the regular clergy, An intractable and revengeful spirit, Political restlessness, Vain glory, Uncharitableness, Profaneness, Uncleanness, The spirit of family discord, Freakishness and distraction, and Insanity, it has the tendency to betray its votaries into every irregularity, and to plunge them into every vice.[34]

Polwhele's emphasis on vain glory, freakishness and distraction links his critique of Methodism to conventional attacks against the tendency of fashion to appeal to women's vanity. His list also chimes with several of Lady Delacour's symptoms, especially knavery, political restlessness, the spirit of family discord, freakishness, distraction and insanity.[35]

Over the course of the novel, until the revelation that Lady Delacour's breast is healthy underneath its surface bruising and subsequent mistreatment by both herself and quack doctors, Edgeworth paints a picture of the connecting ways in which fashionable femininity is beset by associated sexual, physical and mental health problems. Significantly, the most serious threat to Lady Delacour's health stems from her reading: her flirtation with Methodism is literary in nature, underscoring the deleterious effects books were thought to have on a woman's health at the time. Several critics have noted the range, depth and breadth of literary references Edgeworth makes in *Belinda*, with Heather Macfadyen focusing on Lady Delacour's fashionable reading.[36] I argue that Edgeworth's engagement with health, fashion and artifice combine in her metatextual manoeuvring towards the end of the novel. Lady Delacour constantly draws the reader's attention to the artificiality of novelistic conventions, linking these to the artifices implicated in representing the healthiness of the female body, particularly through medicine, dress and cosmetics. Having traced Lady Delacour's fashionable diseases in terms of sexuality, physicality and psychology, I turn now to discussing her fashionably self-conscious engagement with texts, before drawing these themes together in her treatment of Clarence Hervey's ward, Virginia St Pierre.

The connections Edgeworth makes between fashion, artifice and metatextuality in her representation of Lady Delacour's instability become particularly apparent in her references to the political philosopher William Godwin, notorious by the end of the eighteenth century for his controversial views on government and religion. Caricatures of Godwin appear in a series of texts by women writers at this time, from his former friend Amelia Opie's *roman á clef*, *Adeline Mowbray*, in which he appears as the Wollstonecraftian heroine's philosophical lover Glenmurray, to Elizabeth Hamilton's *Memoirs of Modern Philosophers*, in which Mr Myope quotes copiously from Godwin's texts. Whereas Deborah Weiss debates Belinda and Harriet's positions as 'true' and 'false' female philosophers in 'The Extraordinary Ordinary Belinda', I focus on Lady Delacour's role as Godwinian mentor, like Glenmurray in *Adeline Mowbray* or Mr Myope in *Modern Philosophers*, marked by her scattered references to Godwin's texts and her status as unreliable role model for Belinda.[37] Weiss argues that Freke takes on all of the negative associations of the counter-revolutionary iteration of the female philosopher figure which allows Edgeworth to portray Belinda sympathetically as an Enlightenment-style female philosopher, shorn of the figure's threatening revolutionary overtones. I agree with Weiss's argument, which further works for the way in which Hamilton depicts her anti-heroine, the ultra-feminist Bridgetina Botherim in opposition to her domestic heroine Harriet Orwell. My focus on Lady Delacour shows how Edgeworth reintroduces subversive elements of revolutionary philosophy into the novel, which she elsewhere sanitizes with her characterization of Belinda as a 'safe' female philosopher. Lady Delacour's subversiveness resides in her increasingly confident questioning of conventional representations of women's health.

Lady Delacour refers to Godwin's writing explicitly at two points in the novel, both moments of crisis in her relationship with Belinda. The first appears at the end of the chapter entitled 'Jealousy', concluding in Belinda's decision to leave the Delacour household and take up her invitation to stay with the Percivals. Belinda decides to leave her friend after Lady Delacour accuses her of seducing Lord Delacour in an attempt to become his second wife after Lady Delacour's death. In order to conceal her real pain at Belinda's departure, Lady Delacour appears '[f]resh rouged, and elegantly dressed ... performing her part to a brilliant audience in the drawing room, when Belinda entered' in order to leave the house. Lady Delacour, 'turning carelessly towards her', asks Belinda:

> Miss Portman ... where do you buy your rouge? Lady Singleton, would you rather at this moment be mistress of the philosopher's stone, or have a patent for rouge that will come and go like miss Portman's? A propos, have you read St Leon?' her ladyship was running on to a fresh train of ideas, when a footman announced the arrival of lady Anne Percival's carriage; and miss Portman rose to depart.[38]

Seeing that Belinda is really going to leave, Lady Delacour's performance breaks down and she begs her to stay; Belinda is only capable of repeating 'Adieu!' before hurrying out of the house 'with the strongest feeling of compassion for this unhappy woman, but with an unaltered sense of the propriety and necessity of her own firmness'.[39] Lady Delacour's speech plays upon Belinda's real blushes, deliberately mistaking them for a make-up which gives the appearance of eternal youth, before noticing that Belinda's blushes 'come and go'. Lady Delacour's reference to *St Leon* signifies at once her movement onto a different set of ideas and suggests to the reader a set of connections between her character and Godwin's flawed narrator: personal nobility corrupted by social mores – St Leon is nearly destroyed by gambling, Lady Delacour by fashion; and their egotism both damages their physical and mental health and fractures the family unit.

Lady Delacour's use of St Leon further complicates Edgeworth's exploration of female nature versus artifice. By teasingly misreading Belinda's real blushes as make-up, Lady Delacour ironically connects Belinda's youthful inexperience with not only St Leon's more cynical pursuit of the philosopher's stone but her own jaded concern to disguise the aging process. Her comments to Lady Singleton hint at women's worries about aging, and also suggest Lady Delacour's, and Edgeworth's, critique of societal double standards: society demands that women conform to an image of youthful naturalness which becomes more and more untenable with age, finally depending on the artifice it seems to scorn. Lady Delacour's fears about aging, therefore, link Edgeworth's focus on women's health – the increased frailty and social exclusion which attends the aging process – with her engagement with fashion, which seeks to disguise aging by advocating the perpetual youthfulness which Edgeworth hints is as much a fantasy as the philosopher's stone. Edgeworth's intertextual allusion to Godwin's 1799 novel forges a series of connections between the two writers, using Godwin's critique of the way in which social pressures fracture individual relationships with families to explore a more feminine quandary. In this way, Lady Delacour functions as a much more positive representative of a Godwinian mentor than either Glenmurray or Mr Myope. Both *St. Leon* and *Belinda* partake in liberal political and aesthetic strategies seeking to reformulate revolutionary philosophy in a post-revolutionary context. Both texts aim to reform reading habits, social norms and, in Edgeworth's novel especially, gendered preconceptions, to a progressive agenda against conservative demands for unquestioning loyalist obedience in the context of the Napoleonic wars.

In the chapter called 'Reconciliation', Edgeworth reunites Lady Delacour with both her estranged husband and Belinda, showing how Lady Delacour struggles to reconcile Belinda with her suitor Clarence Hervey, particularly his mysterious relationship with Virginia St Pierre. Lady Delacour shows Belinda the letters she has received from Clarence during his equally mysterious journey through Dorset and Devonshire. Focusing on his description of a happy marriage, designed to encourage Lady Delacour's rapprochement with her Lord, she comments that:

> I take it all in good part, because, to do Clarence justice, he describes the joys of domestic Paradise in such elegant language, that he does not make me sick. In short, my dear Belinda, to finish my panegyric, as it has been said of some other epistles, if ever there were letters calculated to make you fall in love with the writer of them, these are they.[40]

These last lines deliberately echo Godwin's assessment of Wollstonecraft's *Letters from Sweden*: 'If ever there was a book calculated to make a man in love with its author, this appears to me to be the book'.[41] Edgeworth plays with gender categories here, allowing Lady Delacour to perform Godwin's role of seduced critic and placing Hervey in Wollstonecraft's position as seductive letter writer. Edgeworth's playful, literary allusions to Godwin here differentiate her from both Hamilton's critique of Godwinian political philosophy as dangerous and damaging to established social structures in *Modern Philosophers* and Opie's satire of Godwin's anti-marital arguments in *Adeline Mowbray*. Aligning Lady Delacour with Godwin reveals her radical inheritance, underscoring her threat to social structures of stability and making Edgeworth's decision to redeem her at the end of the novel intriguing. On the other hand, Lady Delacour seems distinctly anti-Godwinian. Godwin argued for sincerity, candour and a strict adherence to truth throughout his writing career, whereas Lady Delacour seems to value 'unhealthy' artifice above 'healthy' nature: throughout the novel, Lady Delacour both argues for the importance of and maintains a fashionable façade and questions the naturalness of social prescriptions on the healthiness of a woman's body. In the end, what Edgeworth offers in Lady Delacour is her reimagining of the Godwinian hero, unreliable, complex and conflicted, as heroine – reenergizing the revolutionary nostalgia in Godwin's portrait of St Leon's dutiful, domestic, dying wife Marguerite de Damville in the more active, compelling and finally elusive Lady Delacour.

Although Edgeworth reveals the social costs of this artificiality – Lady Delacour's happy exterior belies a profoundly miserable woman – the novel remains as suspicious as Lady Delacour is of naturalness. Clarence Hervey's desire to educate his ward, Virginia St Pierre, as a natural woman is revealed to be wishful thinking – a male sexual fantasy – which leads to a distinct decline in her mental and physical health. Hervey draws his educational theories from Rousseau, tellingly described by Edgeworth as an 'eloquent' writer, highlighting Rousseau's fashionable caché by the end of the eighteenth century. Throughout the chapter revealing Virginia's mysterious background, Edgeworth stresses how much Hervey is influenced not only by fashionable educational theory but by wider fashion in literature at the time, for example, he changes his ward's name from Rachel to Virginia after the exemplary fictional heroine of Henri Bernardin de St Pierre's *Paul et Virginie* (1787), which, as Edgeworth makes clear, reveals the fictive nature of Hervey's enterprise.

Hervey refuses to educate Virginia about the fashionable world, keeping her in splendid isolation, and, significantly, ignorance. In this isolation, Virginia reads romances which encourage her febrile imagination to invent her own sexual fantasy surrounding a mysterious figure from her past, then to feel guilty for not being attracted to the neglectful Hervey. Although Hervey manages to keep Virginia secluded from fashionable society, his growing boredom with her leads her to, ironically, find solace in just the sort of fashionable reading matter which Hervey has both censored her from accessing and accessed himself to fashion her. In trying to create a 'natural' woman, Hervey only succeeds in fashioning a doubly fashionable woman: formed firstly from Hervey's Rousseauvian pedagogy and secondly by her own taste for popular romance. Virginia's fictive development leads her to the brink of ill health. Tormented by nightmares which testify to her guilt about the lack of attraction she feels towards Hervey – one of which ends with him berating her as 'Perfidious, *ungrateful* Virginia! you are the cause of my death!'– Virginia sinks into depression, characterized by dejection, tearfulness and aversion to Hervey.[42]

Both Hervey and Virginia, although neither of them are attracted to the other, feel duty bound to marry each other through misunderstanding: Hervey because he feels responsible for Virginia's passive state of childish ignorance and Virginia because she feels it to be Hervey's expectation of her. Lady Delacour is instrumental in separating the two mismatched non-lovers, declaring to Belinda, the real object of Hervey's affections, 'This Virginia! O, how I hate her! I am sure Clarence cannot love her'.[43] When Belinda upbraids her for hating a woman she has never met, Lady Delacour responds, 'Oh, I know what she must be ... a soft, sighing, dying damsel, who puts bullfinches in her bosom'.[44] Edgeworth adds to Lady Delacour's knowing caricature of Virginia's clichéd status as an ideal woman by having her 'anxious to carry away with her but a little bullfinch' on Hervey's first adoption of her.[45] Lady Delacour self-consciously orchestrates Virginia's reunion with both her father, whose bout of madness also taints with suspicion the healthiness of his daughter, and Captain Sunderland, the original behind her romantic fantasies, which leads to Hervey's declaration of love for Belinda.

Lady Delacour takes on an explicitly metatextual role in the novel's final scenes, asking the other characters, the reader of the novel and perhaps Edgeworth herself: 'shall I finish the novel for you?',[46] and concluding by manipulating the various characters into a deliberately staged tableau:

> 'Yes', said her ladyship; 'it is so difficult, as the critic says, to get lovers off upon their knees. Now I think of it, let me place you all in proper attitudes for stage effect. What signifies being happy, unless we appear so? Captain Sunderland – kneeling with Virginia, if you please, sir, at her father's feet. You in the act of giving your blessing, Mr. Hartley. Mrs. Ormond clasps her hands with joy – nothing can be better than that, madam – I give you infinite credit for the attitude. Clarence, you have a right to Belinda's hand, and may kiss it too. Nay, miss Portman, it is the rule of the stage. Now, where's my lord Delacour? He should be embracing me, to show that we are reconciled. Ha! here he comes. Enter lord Delacour, with little Helena in his hand. Very well! a good start of surprise, my lord. Stand still, pray, you cannot be better than you are. Helena, my love, do not let go your father's hand. There! quite pretty and natural! Now, lady Delacour, to show that she is reformed, comes forward to address the audience with a moral – a moral! – yes,
>
> Our *tale* contains a *moral*, and, no doubt,
> You all have wit enough to find it out'.[47]

As Egenolf points out, although Lady Delacour gestures towards her new, willing subordination to her husband, she actually commands him to stay with his daughter, remaining centre stage herself. By doing so, she 'avoids the controlling domestic structure of the scene and unsettles the familial stability of this tableau vivant'.[48] Contrary to Greenfield's reading of Lady Delacour as inhabiting the role of 'proper lady' in this conclusion, she escapes from the domestic plot of Edgeworth's finale, leaving the text's anxieties open to the reader's own interpretation. Belinda and Harriet, as contrasting representations of the female philosopher figure, are sidelined in this final scene in favour of Lady Delacour, offering Edgeworth's alternative reading of the thinking woman, dominant, contradictory and performative.

3 TRANSFORMING THE BODY POLITIC: FOOD REFORM AND FEMINISM IN NINETEENTH-CENTURY BRITAIN

Sarah Richardson

The idea of the state as a corporeal being – the body politic – became increasingly gendered during the nineteenth century. Two major pieces of legislation in the 1830s, the 1832 Reform Act and the 1835 Municipal Corporations Act, vested the right to vote, and therefore the right to citizenship, in 'male persons'. This has led many historians to argue that politics was effectively 'masculinized' during this period.[1] However, Victorian radical women challenged their exclusion from the public sphere and questioned if the legislative changes had created a healthier state. In arguing for a stronger, fitter state they drew on contemporary debates about alternative forms of medicine and diet. In both areas, power and control would be removed from a largely masculine political and medical establishment, and placed in the hands of women. This essay considers the contribution of two female activists in the field of dietary reform and feminist politics: Anna Kingsford and Annie Cobden-Sanderson. These women were part of a wider campaign to feminize and to democratize the body and the state.

The metaphor of the state as a body politic was appropriated and reinvented by generations of reformers. Seventeenth- and eighteenth-century political theorists, including Hobbes, Locke and Rousseau, employed the image creatively in their interpretations of the source of political authority.[2] The famous frontispiece to Hobbes's *Leviathan* vividly illustrates the concept. The etching by Abraham Bosse depicts a gargantuan crowned figure emerging from the landscape; his head and hands have recognizable features, but his body is comprised of hundreds of tiny figures, representing the embodiment of the state. The notion of the state as a living body, a voluntary association of individuals, encouraged discussion about the health and vitality of the nation, as well as suggestions of possible remedies. This model, did not, as has been suggested by Kevin Sharpe and Steven Zwicker, lose its potency with the bloodshed and terror of the French Revolution.[3] Instead, as Roy Porter has demonstrated, new representations of the body and of disease in the early nineteenth century led to a resurgence of caricatures and political satire portraying government and governors in human form.[4] The close proximity of the legislation on Catholic Emancipation and electoral reform from 1828–32 and the passage of the 1832 Anatomy Act engendered a plethora of images linking body and state.[5] William Heath's 1829 print, 'Burking Poor Old Mrs Constitution, Aged 141' and the sketch, 'Burkeing the Constitution of E–g–d!!!!' drew parallels between the passage of the Catholic Emancipation Act and the activities of the notorious Burke and Hare anatomy murders. The constitution was portrayed in human female form being suffocated by the Duke of Wellington and Sir Robert Peel, the architects of the legislation. In a similar vein, Robert Seymour's series of sketches on the Reform Bill for McLean's *Monthly Sheet of Caricatures or the Looking Glass* in 1832 directly associated the anatomists with the tortuous passage of the Act. One print, 'Burkers Exulting over their Victim' shows members of the House of Lords, depicted as Burke and Hare, sitting on a chest containing the 'Reform Bill'. In the second, 'The Victim Reanimated', the Bill springs from the chest as the 'Burkers' scurry away. The satires chart the attempt by the Lords to throw out the Reform Bill, an attempt which ultimately failed with the passage of a third version in December 1831. The vulnerability of the state was compared to the frail victims of Burke and Hare; the state's body could literally be snatched away by corrupt and unscrupulous politicians.

As the nineteenth century progressed, discussions focused less on competing versions of the body politic, and turned instead to debates about whose bodies should be represented by the polity. Most contemporary commentators assumed the state was white, male and middle class. This was put most pithily by the American intellectual Orestes Brownson:

> Now political equality between man is represented by universal suffrage. Universal suffrage, necessarily recognizes each man as a member of the body politic by virtue, not of his possessions, his endowments, his accidents, but by virtue of his manhood.[6]

Brownson saw no tension in his use of the term 'universal suffrage' and the limitation of this privilege to men. Indeed, in his view, membership of the body politic was a signifier of manliness. Feminist campaigners struggled with the paradox that 'equal rights' could be denied to women and other groups. Thus, a petitioner, Mary Smith of Stanmore in Yorkshire, argued that the 1832 Reform Act should include female taxpayers as well as male. As women were liable to all the punishments of the law, they ought to have a voice in the making of them.[7] As Joan Scott has argued, in the context of the French Revolution, citizenship was assumed to depend on the physical characteristics of the male human body and this problematized claims by women to be full and active citizens in the liberal state.[8] Campaigners thus presented the condition of the state as the problem. By limiting the political nation to propertied men, the constitution was ailing, unhealthy, damaged and in need of healing to be restored to full vigour. For example, the activist Millicent Garret Fawcett, commenting on the tactics of militant suffragettes (which she condemned), nevertheless put the responsibility firmly on the shoulders of politicians:

> Statesmen are the physicians of the body politic. When things go wrong, when, for instance, women, who are by nature gentle and refined, take to conduct which is condemned … these disorders are symptoms of a social disease to the cure of which statesmen should apply themselves.[9]

Many women's rights campaigners, however, rejected the idea that the unhealthy state could be cured either by the ministrations of politicians or by recourse to doctors and conventional medicine, for they were considered to be part of the problem. As Claire Brock argues in this volume, the medical profession was overwhelmingly male, and women activists regarded doctors as agents of the establishment. The lack of control women had over medical interventions on their own bodies mirrored their limited rights in the public sphere. Feminist outrage against what they viewed as politicians' and physicians' violation of female bodies was at its height during the campaigns against the Contagious Diseases Acts where women suspected of prostitution could be forcibly detained and subjected to brutal internal examinations.[10] The overwhelmingly male state and medical profession colluded to target and abuse vulnerable women, rather than the men using the prostitutes. In light of all this, many campaigners concluded that the solution to a healthy polity comprising of vigorous, fit citizens would not be supplied by the male-dominated medical profession. For many activists, the health of their own body and that of the state was dependent upon them wresting control from the authorities and taking over the management of their own well-being. One of the key elements that emerged in this struggle between the establishment and women's rights activists centred on that vital element for survival: food.

Historians engaging in debates about the links between women's rights and the 'embodiment of resistance' tend to focus their attention on militant suffragists' campaign of hunger strikes.[11] The refusal of food was a weapon against an oppressive and unreasonable state. The response by the authorities to institute forcible feeding was portrayed in suffrage memoirs as violations of women's bodies. Yet, the focus on the hunger strike – an exercise in control and self-discipline by the refusal of nourishment – fails to take account of the backstory to the many and varied connections between food, feminism and political reform. The Food Reform Movement emerged in Germany in the 1820s, and, as Kathryn Gleadle has cogently argued, was quickly adopted by British radicals keen to accompany political change with a democratization of the 'care and feeding of the body'.[12] Food and health reform formed essential components of female public identities around the time of the 1832 Reform Act leading to the politicization of the household as a site for activism.[13] Dietetic reformers encompassed a diverse group of campaigners: vegetarians, vegans, fruitarians, schools meals activists and, by extension, those against cruelty to animals, including anti-vivisectionists. There were strong links between the personnel of these movements and of wider female political reform organizations. This essay examines the important connections between the food reformers and women's rights activists in the nineteenth century through, as alluded to above, the lens of the work of two key crusaders: Anna Kingsford (1846–88) and Annie Cobden-Sanderson (1853–1926). Their significant, but under-appreciated, contribution will be utilized to demonstrate the interweaving of issues of women's health and feminism in this period. Food reform enabled women to highlight fundamental issues about their participation in the public sphere, their subjugation and lack of a voice on civic matters by evoking similarities between their own treatment and that of animals. Moreover, in making these connections, they were drawing upon a rich discourse which had long linked corruption and decay in the political establishment with unhealthy and unbalanced diets. Purity in the body politic depended upon democracy and simplicity; similar virtues could be applied to the health of the physical body.

Anna Kingsford was an unconventional writer, physician, spiritualist, lecturer and radical campaigner.[14] Although suffering from debilitating bouts of ill health, she nevertheless pursued training for a medical degree in France, since women were excluded from British universities until the end of the century. Her studies had been prompted by a desire to learn more about medical research, as a result of a growing interest in the anti-vivisection movement. She professed to have completed her degree without recourse to vivisection. Kingsford became a vegetarian in 1870, inspired by her brother, and for her dissertation considered the medical, economic and social benefits of a vegetable diet. She also viewed herself as a 'political woman', albeit one who appreciated female 'charm and gentleness', regretting the tendency to reject the aesthetic in the 'zeal for the serious and useful'. In her first editorial, for the *Lady's Own Paper*, subtitled a journal of 'progress, taste, and thought', which she purchased in 1872 in order to pursue a career as a journalist, she noted: 'Some years ago we were exclusively domestic; now we are inclined to be exclusively politic'.[15] The first edition of the periodical demonstrated this mix of concerns with both public affairs and domestic issues: it included articles on women's education, the revision of the Russian Bible and the art of fine dress. The second issue reflected Kingsford's growing concern about the practice of vivisection with an article by Henry J. Bigelow, Professor of Surgery at Harvard, and a letter on the subject from the feminist journalist and campaigner, Frances Power Cobbe. There was also an article by Dr Charles Drysdale on 'Why all educated women should study physiology and hygiene' which concluded that 'little advance can be expected in morality then until our women on a grand scale commence to study the only science which can lead to a sound knowledge of human life, its duties and responsibilities – physiology'.[16] The connection between health, diet and women's contribution to public life were themes that Kingsford would return to throughout her career. However, she also continued to pay attention to the personal and domestic concerns of women, publishing a volume entitled *Health, Beauty, and the Toilet. Letters to Ladies from a Lady Doctor* in 1886. The letters contained practical advice on diet and health but also the 'cosmetic arts' and attention to the 'improvement and preservation of physical grace and good looks' accompanied by relevant medical and scientific references.[17]

Kingsford's first foray into the arena of political debate came with a pamphlet she wrote to support efforts in Parliament to admit women to the municipal and parliamentary franchise. Writing under the pen-name Ninon Kingsford, her *Essay on the Admission of Women to the Parliamentary Franchise* argued that voting would 'give women a higher place in society' and 'lift them from the level of goods and chattels to the position which they ought to occupy, of citizens and of responsible beings'.[18] These points were not particularly novel, forming the main contention of the various women's suffrage societies and petitions that flourished in the late 1860s. However, the bulk of Kingsford's pamphlet was not devoted to making a political case but instead asserting that the cause of women's inferior status in public life lay in their lack of physical exercise. She compared the education of girls unfavourably with that of boys: 'No races, no football, no chase, no merry rompings in the playground, because, forsooth, such games are not fit for young ladies!'. The health and strength of the body were essential to insure 'power and elasticity' to the mind, necessary prerequisites for active citizenship.[19] Although the pamphlet was written before her conversion to vegetarianism and her medical training, she nonetheless considered that women could not lead fulfilled lives and make a proper contribution to society if they were not 'fed and supported with proper nourishment'.[20] Thus, for Kingsford, physical factors were as significant as intellectual or ideological issues in discussions about women's role in public life.

The bulk of Anna Kingsford's publications were on the subject of vegetarianism, including the English translation of her dissertation, which was published in 1881 as *The Perfect Way in Diet*. She drew upon a vast array of evidence and argument to support the adoption of a meat-free regime, enumerating the economic advantages, health benefits and theological justifications. Moreover, threaded throughout was a strong feminist tone and she returned again and again to the particular rewards for women who implemented dietetic reform. These touched on all aspects of their lives including their domestic role, education, employment, and legal and civil rights. Food reform was thus part of a general thrust towards progress in all arenas of public and private life. She asserted that the hostile and male-dominated establishment that had led to the formation of women's rights movements also gave rise to vegetarianism. The concerns mooted about the subjection of women by their male relatives were in a similar vein to those raised about meat-eating; both were considered to be uncivilized and backward. In one lecture, she heralded the dawn of a new era: 'out of the purifying furnace springs the aspirations of the new age, vigorous and strong, full of life and youth and purpose'.[21] This would extend rights to women as well as animals.

Her thesis did not merely emphasize the empowering and emancipatory aspects but also extended the views that she expounded in the *Lady's Own Paper* that science, politics and economy should take account of the aesthetic and beautiful. In *Letters on Pure Diet* which appeared in the *Food Reform Magazine* in 1881–2, she asserted that the case for dietetic reform was not solely scientific but also appealed to intuitional faculties:

> On the one hand we are able to command the advocacy of Comparative Anatomy and Physiology, Chemistry, Hygiene, and Economy Social and Political; on the other, our cause is pleaded by all the arts which beautify life and civilize humanity.[22]

In *Addresses to Vegetarians*, Kingsford noted that the great majority of men classified women as 'housekeepers', whose chief duty was to prepare (or to superintend the preparation of) food. However, the close contact with the slaughterhouse, butcher's shop and dead carcasses made it an occupation 'at once unwomanly, unhuman, and barbarous in the extreme'.[23] Thus, she cunningly subverted the dominant 'separate spheres' ideology: the kitchen was no place for the gentler sex if it brought them into contact with the blood, guts and brutality of the slaughter of animals for food. In her lecture 'Some Aspects of the Vegetarian Question' she also claimed that the vegetarian system was 'pre-eminently calculated to rescue women from the drudgery that threatens them in respect of the culinary art' and was therefore a fundamental aspect of female emancipation. She argued that the simple, wholesome vegetarian diet required less than half the 'hard toil and anxiety' of cooking with meat.[24]

Her reasoning was fully referenced and illustrated with pertinent examples. In *A Lecture on Food* which was delivered to the female students of Girton College, Cambridge in 1882 she prioritized the economic benefits of a meat-free diet, maintaining that a shilling spent on oatmeal, peas, lentils or beans would purchase as much nutriment as five shillings spent on meat. She referred to the temperance campaigner, William Hoyle's text, *Our National Resources, and How they are Wasted* to calculate that if the six million families of the United Kingdom reduced their consumption of meat by a pound's weight per week, it would save over ten million pounds a year.[25] She argued that girls should be instructed in the 'science and resources' of housekeeping with special reference made to the art of vegetarian cookery and of 'making savoury and appetizing dishes out of inexpensive materials' in order to improve the health and income of the poor. In a further lecture, she turned to the question of health, drawing on statistics from the *Science of Health Journal*. Again, she foregrounded the impact on women's lives. As four-fifths of the cost of medicine and medical advice was spent on female and infant health, and nine-tenths of nursing and care of sick children was undertaken by women, a simpler 'hygienic' diet would be of primary benefit to women.[26] Perhaps her most controversial claim linking the status of women with a carnivorous diet came in her book, *The Best Food for Man*. Here she claimed that the amount of land devoted to rearing animals for food led directly to 'poverty, dirt, squalor, drink, crime'. But more heinous than those evils, it resulted in the 'enforced exile' of agricultural labourers and the 'consequent surplus of a helpless female population of a million souls'.[27] She thus tapped into the widespread anxiety by social reformers concerning the 'redundant woman' question which had been quantified by the decennial censuses from 1851 onwards. However, her allegation that the surplus of single women (as well as the other social evils listed) was directly caused by a meat-eating diet is extreme, and she does not attempt to substantiate the assertion with any evidence. It does, however, tap into the anxieties of the establishment who viewed the sexual imbalance of the population as a threat. These concerns had been voiced most articulately by the journalist and reformer, W. R. Greg in an article entitled 'Why are Women Redundant?' in 1862. His solution was to encourage 400,000 women to emigrate to the colonies where there was a surplus of men. A response by Frances Power Cobbe entitled 'What Shall We Do with our Old Maids?' questioned why there was no similar apprehension about the 25 per cent of men who remained single.[28] Of course, if unmarried women were admitted to the franchise and thus the body politic, their numbers were such that they had the potential to make a significant impact.

Anna Kingsford paid equal attention to female emancipation in the public and private spheres. In her lectures and publications, she extended ideas about the radicalization of the home and household which were prevalent in the discourse of the food reformers of the 1840s. As Kathryn Gleadle identified in her scrutiny of the early vegetarian movement, the reconciliation of domesticity with politics was an essential strategy for women to express their opinions in an era where female participation in the public sphere was limited.[29] Kingsford also pioneered many of the contentions that were to found the basis of the more formal links between the vegetarian and women's suffrage movements, which Leah Leneman considers were cemented in the 1890s.[30] Her contribution was significant, not merely due to the quantity of lectures she delivered and the extent of her published work, but also because of her medical and scientific training which provided an empirical foundation which other writers could draw upon. The key word, for Kingsford, in the achievement of the 'perfect way' in diet and in politics, was 'purity'. She advocated that the proper and natural food for man was uncooked, therefore she survived mainly on fruit and nuts, eating only a little cooked vegetarian food.[31] A pure diet and a healthy body should be based on austere simplicity. Purity, and the elimination of corruption, in the public domain depended on the full inclusion and emancipation of women.

The individual whose life and work perhaps most comprehensively summarizes the connections between food, feminism and the body politic was Annie Cobden-Sanderson. She was one of five surviving daughters of the noted free trade politician, Richard Cobden.[32] More radical than her sisters, she joined the Independent Labour Party, was a member of the National Union of Women Suffrage Societies (NUWSS) and later, the more militant Women's Social and Political Union (WSPU). She had been a vegetarian since the age of twenty, and an interest in food reform underpinned much of her activism. In 1906, she was arrested along with nine other members of the WSPU after a disturbance in the lobby of the House of Commons. The forcible detention of Cobden's daughter triggered a wave of public sympathy for the disproportionate reaction to the demonstration. In her account of the women's suffrage movement, Sylvia Pankhurst acknowledged the important of the Cobden connection. She asserted that Cobden-Sanderson's arrest 'caused consternation in Government circles; for though Mrs Cobden-Sanderson had joined the ILP, the fact that she was Cobden's daughter would be remembered in the country'.[33] George Bernard Shaw, a fellow vegetarian and activist, in an excoriating letter to *The Times* also spoke of the ignominy for the establishment in arresting and locking up 'the charming and interesting' Annie Cobden-Sanderson:

> The peril [to Britain] today wears a darker, deadlier aspect. Ten women – ten petticoated, long-stockinged, corseted females have hurled themselves on the British Houses of Parliament. Desperate measures are necessary ... To the immortal glory of our Metropolitan Police they did not blanch. They carried the lady out even as they carried Bradlaugh. But they did not dare to leave her at large as they left him. They held on to her like grim death until they had her safe under bolt and bar ... we might, perhaps, venture to let Mrs Cobden-Sanderson and her friends out ... We should still look ridiculous, but at least the lady would not be a martyr ... Will not the Home Secretary rescue us from a ridiculous, an intolerable, and incidentally a revoltingly spiteful and unmanly situation?[34]

Shaw considered that the violence used against the women was far greater than that employed against any male protestors. However, ultimately this extreme reaction emasculated and undermined the authorities. The women were released early from their sentences, just before a crucial by-election in Huddersfield.

Although Cobden-Sanderson was imprisoned before the suffragettes began implementing the tactic of hunger strikes to publicize their cause further, she nevertheless suffered immense privation in prison, the more so because of her vegetarian diet. In an open letter to the press, her husband detailed her treatment including twenty-three hours of solitary confinement per day and meals of dry bread, tea or cocoa and potatoes.[35] Millicent Garrett Fawcett, who remained friendly with Cobden-Sanderson in spite of her defection to the WSPU, visited her in prison, and was appalled that her dinner consisted of three potatoes, the prison authorities being ill-equipped to deal with a vegetarian prisoner.[36] Cobden-Sanderson resisted her harsh treatment whilst in prison, and continued to raise awareness about the poor conditions once free. Her cell was infested by cockroaches so she complained to the prison governor, but refused the offer of a move, recognizing that whoever later occupied her cell would face the same conditions.[37] On her release, she wrote a series of letters to the newspapers exposing the poor environment in prison, including the freezing temperatures on the hospital wards. Her motivation was to improve the treatment of women prisoners but also to draw attention to the fact that they were incarcerated as a result of legislation enacted by an entirely male government and judiciary:

> In the name of all women who are in prison, and in prison for disobeying laws which they have no voice in making and no power to alter, I protest against the present inhuman system of our prisons, of which this is only one example.[38]

She concluded that 'the fulfilment of the Law of Prisons is morally worse than the infringement of the laws which leads to them', placing guilt firmly on the shoulders of Parliament.[39] Her solution was not to introduce women prison officers, who could only follow the orders of their male superiors, but the engagement of a female commissioner who had the power to effect improvements. For Cobden-Sanderson though, institutional change could only be realized if it was accompanied by physical, bodily improvements. She argued that,

> in order to make people better you must attend to their physical conditions, and provide them with plenty of fresh air, sunlight, and clear water, and bring cleanliness and self-respect to the body and pity and sympathy to the soul.

Food was an essential element of the health and well-being of the prisoners and of the institution itself. She hoped that prison doctors would be instructed that 'it is not only the suffragist or passive resister who needs wholesome food'.[40] It was fitting, given Cobden-Sanderson's emphasis on the importance of food to politics, that on her release from prison, a banquet was held in her honour, hosted by Millicent Garrett Fawcett. The banquet was announced by the Court Circular in *The Times*, and was held at the Savoy: a symbolic show of strength by the women's suffrage movement to the metropolitan establishment.[41]

In her juvenile diaries and letters Cobden-Sanderson had expressed concern for animals, nature and the environment, causes which forged her early political identity. In her brief memoir explaining how she became vegetarian, it was clear that animal rights activism formed part of her belief system infusing all aspects of her ideological outlook.[42] Food reform continued to be an important strand to her political pursuits throughout her career. In 1908 she was instrumental in establishing the New Food Reform Movement with Sarah Grand, and fellow vegetarians Charlotte Despard, Beatrice Webb and Seebohm Rowntree. The professed aim of the movement was 'to enlighten public opinion on matters of diet' and 'to point out the dangers of our present system of food supply'.[43] Eugenics and social Darwinism formed a key theme of the movement. One supporter argued that vegetarianism was a natural consequence of the evolution of the human race which was moving away from barbarous practices such as the slaughter and consumption of animals. A vegetarian diet had social benefits, with followers more open to progress and exercising higher moral values. He concluded that:

> Great and far-reaching will be the effects of the Nation's adoption of a pure and bloodless diet – there will be better health, great intelligence, higher ideas, deeper spirituality, and in addition to all these benefits there are questions of national importance which will thus find their solution.[44]

Food reformers, like Cobden-Sanderson, believed diet could solve many of the problems of the age, and also that women were best placed to tackle these. She was particularly interested in the question of children's food. In a paper she wrote for the *British Health Review* entitled 'Housekeeping for the Nation's Children' she echoed some of the eugenicist sentiments of the food reformers, arguing that 'we must look to the change in diet as the chief cause for the present degeneracy'.[45] Her ideas were in line with many on the left, particularly the Fabians Sidney and Beatrice Webb, who were the leading socialist promoters of 'national efficiency'.[46] In her paper, Cobden-Sanderson suggested five dinner menus which would solve the problem, most containing a small amount of fish or meat but also reliant on a large amount of root vegetables, fruit, wholemeal bread and porridge. She suggested using the 'less refined' kind of bread which should be made crusty by rebaking in the oven, serving to 'cleanse the teeth, and at the same time oblige the children to eat slowly, and properly masticate their food'.[47]

Cobden-Sanderson crusaded against the traditionally heavy, rich meat diet of the period arguing that it was wasteful, harmful to health and bad for the digestion. In 1908 she spoke at a conference calling for the scientific feeding of schoolchildren organized in response to the introduction of school meals by the National Food Reform Association. She reiterated her view of the danger of the food provided for children by local authorities: 'Children in elementary schools had long been underfed. But there was now a danger of their being overfed in the schools by being given food which was too heavy for them.'[48] She later elaborated her views on the need for a scientific approach to the feeding of schoolchildren in a pamphlet she wrote with Margaret McMillan for the Independent Labour Party entitled *London's Children. How to Feed Them and How Not to Feed Them*. Here, she contended, 'The feeding of children ... is a NATIONAL question, which has for its object the building up of a strong and healthy race; and the child, and not the education of the parent, must see the object of our solicitude'.[49] Cobden-Sanderson's emphasis on the practicalities of feeding the poor schoolchildren of London was underpinned by her strong ideology that a healthy diet was at the heart of political regeneration.[50] Thus the focus on school meals had a far wider objective, that of transforming national politics. This was also a feminist agenda: it turned a traditional female role (caring for children) into a political concern with national reach. The establishment was charged with failing to nurture the nation's most precious resource: its people. The practical activities of campaigners such as McMillan and Cobden-Sanderson aimed to demonstrate that women were aware of the key social and economic challenges of the age, and knew how to resolve them.

Annie Cobden-Sanderson linked her campaigns for more nutritious diets for working-class children and vegetarianism with her activism in other political movements including the extension of the franchise. However, her enthusiasm for vegetarianism also attracted criticism from her friends who accused her of neglecting more important political matters. William Morris wrote to his wife Jane that Cobden-Sanderson 'is a very unregenerate person with a furious fad towards vegetarianism, in which I see no harm, if it didn't swallow up more important matters'.[51] However, there is little evidence that Annie Cobden-Sanderson's activism was in any way diminished by her championing of food reform. She continued to take a prominent role in the suffrage movement before the war, appearing in court on more than one occasion, and narrowly avoiding imprisonment again in 1909.[52] She maintained a creative approach to her campaigns, establishing tax resistance organizations both to lobby for women's suffrage and to protest against the Insurance Tax which she claimed unfairly burdened the working class.[53] In 1905 she was a founder of the 'Right to Work' committee convened by the Independent Labour Party.[54] The campaign organized several deputations to Parliament and in 1909 Cobden-Sanderson, along with a number of other prominent women socialists including Charlotte Despard and Dora Montefiore, headed a procession of the wives and children of the London unemployed.[55] She also supported the strike in Piccadilly by waitresses who were campaigning for better pay and working conditions.[56] But perhaps the issue that was closest to her heart was the revival of her father's interest in land reform with the objective of freeing land from feudal ownership and redistributing it to the wider population.[57] Again, this was important for Cobden-Sanderson, because she viewed the limited ownership of land, the majority of the country owned by only 2,500 people, as one factor that caused poverty and poor nutritional standards in the masses. In 1909, she wrote a pamphlet, published by the Independent Labour Party with a foreword by Keir Hardie, entitled *Richard Cobden and the Land of the People*.[58] With close reference to Cobden's own speeches and letters, she outlined the connections between free trade and land redistribution. Recognizing that Cobden had put his faith for reform in the middling classes, she sought to extend his vision by harnessing the power of the working classes to the cause of land reform. She linked this with a call for 'political freedom' which would give men and women the right to vote thus opening up to them 'the intellectual outlook which must be the foundation of a civilized state'.[59] In June 1909, she hosted a public meeting at Midhurst in Sussex, the Cobden family home, with the objective of inaugurating the movement for the public ownership of land. Keir Hardie addressed the crowd contending that if the land of this country was divided into smallholdings of five or twenty-five acres, enough foodstuffs could be produced to make the country independent of foreigners.[60] Cobden-Sanderson thus harnessed her father's legacy to the socialist cause. She elaborated her views in a newspaper interview given in 1904 to the *Daily Chronicle* asserting that her father, had he lived, 'would have gone further than merely freeing the food of the people – he would have freed the land'.[61]

The two case studies of Anna Kingsford and Annie Cobden-Sanderson demonstrate how the advocating of a vegetarian, vegan or fructarian diet was fundamental to their feminism. Although Anna Kingsford was an early campaigner for female enfranchisement, she became estranged from the mainstream women's rights movement, perhaps because she gave equal weight to women's role within the household. However, she never lost her fervent feminist beliefs, writing to her friend, Florence Fenwick Miller, towards the end of her life:

> I think, of all your *Lady's Pictorial* papers, I like best those in which you showed by the example of Mendelssohn's sister and Herschel's what women ***might*** be if there were not everlastingly suppressed and bullied into silence. When idiots like ____ tell us women have never been great, that they have been tried and found wanting, and so forth – these little biographies are a pathetically eloquent reply. My heart aches when I read these things, and feel all the pangs of disappointed hope and ambition that women must have suffered.[62]

Both food reform and feminism were essential elements of her practice as one of the first female medical practitioners and also informed her political writing. Annie Cobden-Sanderson was more direct in her feminist beliefs. Her militant actions even led to a short period of imprisonment. However, like Kingsford, she linked dietary reform to transformations in the health of the population and the politics of the nation.

At the end of the nineteenth century, anxiety about the nation's health and well-being were linked with unease that the state was no longer fit for purpose, for example in discussions over the quality of foot soldiers in the Boer War. Heading campaigns which connected both issues were feminist writers, lecturers, medical practitioners and activists. The matters of national importance that they sought to address included the building of a strong and healthy race, solving the land question, feeding the poor and, of course, radically reshaping the political landscape. Food reform enabled women to highlight key issues about their participation in the public sphere, their subjugation and lack of a voice on civic matters by evoking similarities between their own treatment and that of animals. Mona Caird, the novelist and anti-vivisectionist, made this point directly in her strident pamphlet, *Beyond the Pale*:

> it is yet possible, as I have pointed out, to treat women as a class apart, to whom obligations and rights may be arbitrarily apportioned or withheld by the governing sex, – and this is without any sense that a wrong is being done. It is in regard to women and to animals that we see the clearest and grossest survivals from pure savagery.[63]

The overt feminist sentiment was perhaps new. However, links between domestic and health reform and women's role in the national public sphere were not. In correlating concerns about personal health and the state of the nation, women were drawing upon a rich discourse which had long linked corruption and decay in the political establishment with unhealthy and unbalanced diets. Purity in the body politic depended upon democracy and simplicity; similar virtues could be applied to the health of the physical body. A transformation of the body politic was essential to strengthen the physical and moral fibres of the nation, and women were most fitted to deliver this in their role as the traditional overseers of diet and health, and as those untainted by the corruption in the political establishment.

4 STAGNATION OF AIR AND MIND: PICTURING TRAUMA AND MIASMA IN CHARLOTTE BRONTË'S *VILLETTE*

Alexandra Lewis

The pervasive influence of Dr Thomas John Graham's *Modern Domestic Medicine* (1826) in the Brontë household is well known. Patrick Brontë's copy includes extensive marginal annotations relating to his children's health complaints.[1] Like her father, Charlotte took a definite lay interest in medicine, the pseudosciences and the developing field of psychology, and included doctors in her fiction as 'friends offering crucial assistance and understanding'.[2] In *Villette* (1853),[3] the doctor all but replaces the priest in taking confession and endowing revelation intended to lift the spirits. Dr Thomas John Graham and the writers of similar early- to mid-nineteenth-century medical reference works in this way enter Brontë's text in a position of some esteem, through the aptly named fictional practitioner, Dr John Graham Bretton. Though Dr John 'looks in and sees a chamber of torture', however, he 'can neither say nor do much', an acknowledgement of the limitations of his 'art',[4] and of the names and categories assigned in particular to female nervous sufferers. By first considering some of the difficulties experienced in picturing women's mental suffering by, variously, the self-reflexive author of fiction, the fictional 'patient' and the emblematic diagnostician, this chapter then investigates the way theories of miasma, in conjunction with representations of distempered air and storm, are used by Brontë to provide a channel through which images of traumatic disturbance could be explored, beyond the limiting diagnostic categories usually assigned to female sufferers.

Pictures of women in various states of health and decline proliferate in *Villette*: from the 'pale dead nun' painted 'on a panel', to the portrait of Cleopatra – 'ugly' because immodest in abundance – open to female view in a public gallery.[5] It is, however, in the efficacy of characters' self-reading, and self-portraiture – the palimpsest of images stored in the mind – that Brontë's main interest lies. Both the form and content of Brontë's novel are, I argue, centrally concerned with the operations of psychic trauma upon the mind and body of its first-person narrator, Lucy Snowe. How did Charlotte Brontë use fictional autobiography imaginatively to explore questions regarding distinctions between bodily and mental malady, 'masculine' and 'feminine' complaint, and healthy or unhealthy existence?

A wealth of recent interdisciplinary scholarship has begun to examine the complex interface between literature and medicine, illuminating both disease as metaphor and metaphors of disease in Victorian culture.[6] Little attention has been paid, however, to the function of representations of miasma, contagion and epidemic in the Brontës' novels. This is a surprising omission, given not only the prevalence of these concerns within the psychological and medical works with which the novelists were familiar but also, I suggest, the vital relationship between atmosphere and affect, between individual psychology and communal suffering and contagion, through which the Brontës develop what I have elsewhere identified as their innovative poetics of nineteenth-century mental trauma.[7]

This chapter explores the gaps and aporias of traumatic memory at work in *Villette* and the manner in which Brontë manages to represent them with such palpable pain, developing through language and imagery, through her characterization of Lucy Snowe and through the obsessive repetitions of Lucy's life-plot, the picture of a mind labouring under and in many senses frozen or stunted by the lurking presence of unprocessed, unassimilated memories. As part of this consideration, the chapter moves to an examination of the concern with quality of air and of mind worked out in Charlotte Brontë's *Villette*, tracing the ways in which the female narrator's images of pollution, miasma, storm and mental disturbance are negotiated and refigured such that they contribute to a nascent literary psychology of trauma and mnemonic disease. I trace the way dismal, bleak and diseased physical atmospheres are shown by Brontë to infect individual psychic experience – here, the experience of the isolated female – and further explore the effect that these narratives of (mental) contagion and contamination have upon the presentation of women's corporeal experience in *Villette*. This builds into a question I am asking in broader terms: how is the spread of diseased ideas, and of traumatic fragments of the remembered past (both within and between individual minds), inscribed upon the surfaces of bodies and texts in the nineteenth century? Looking beyond phrenological readings, I assess Charlotte Brontë's engagement with scientific and philosophical writings (including works by Robert Burton, George Man Burrows, John Conolly, Thomas John Graham, Henry Holland, J. G. Millingen, James Cowles Prichard and John Reid) on mental instability, female health complaints and prescribed cures, and the effect of unclean and storm-charged air upon the blood and nervous system.

'Something of the Artist's Faculty': Vision, Insight and Partial Representation

Bypassing possibilities for direct authorial or external narrative commentary on Lucy Snowe's perspective on her own fraught history, Brontë creates compelling artistic tensions between that which Lucy is able to see and to narrate within two time frames (the remembered self acting in the past, and the older retrospective subjectivity), and that which she leaves unsaid, whether wilfully or otherwise. I argue that, in her final novel, Brontë creates a narrating mind directed by strong cross-currents, which at once cause Lucy Snowe consciously to attempt to emulate the traumatic obliteration of memory as a kind of coping strategy, and yet ensure that she remains to the last powerfully and unconsciously bound by the very inability to see, relive or relieve the traumatic events of the past, beyond their symbolic, stormy outlines. Notions of traumatic dissociation and flashback, the mechanisms of which continue to generate debate today, are traversed and complicated by Brontë's nuanced account of what James Douglas described in 1839 as the 'sudden resuscitations of past existence': the unexpected resurfacing of memories 'indelibly engraved on the mind'.[8] As such, *Villette* strikes at the heart of the conceptual and rhetorical struggle regarding unconscious cerebration which was to continue to the century's end. Even as William Carpenter described the mind as a wayward horse, capable of overpowering the riding will with its 'independent energy',[9] he sought to minimize the disruptive potential of unconscious activity. From the 1850s on, Carpenter insinuated not only that reflex action of the cerebrum occurred largely as the 'helpmate of reason',[10] but also, crucially, that conscious, moral control could yet be exerted over the uncontrollable inner domain through habituated mental action. Lucy's fictional autobiography navigates a curious course between extremes on the memory spectrum – memory as enabling, controllable power and disabling unconscious pathology – demonstrating the flaws inherent in a rationalist trainable model of the unconscious. She is at once haunted by her past, in the form of nightmares and chains of invasive mental association, and yet unable, even in the final chapter of her written recollections, to give the veiled events of that troubling past full and detailed utterance.

In *Villette*, Lucy Snowe's sufferings are also situated within the prevailing medical models of hypochondriasis and mental illness, represented and diagnosed in the text by Dr John, and indeed partially embraced by Lucy Snowe herself. While using the language of these conditions to construct and explore Lucy's states of mind, Brontë shows how existing diagnoses – like Lucy's own words – fall short of expressing the realities of her intensified yet partial consciousness of personal history and selfhood, occasioned by stunned memory, rather than by an inherently diseased or weakened mind. I suggest that Brontë uses frustrating gaps between available cultural and scientific explanations of women's mental disorders and her central character's painful reality to strain (within and beyond Lucy's more limited awareness) towards a conception of trauma rooted in memory and in those elements of the past which, blocked from conscious view through shock, fear, denial or dissociation, remain inexpressible and therefore potentially insurmountable.

Brontë's narrator begins her autobiography strangely: far from a conventional focus on details of personal memory, the opening scenes of childhood steadfastly insist on the drama of another girl, Paulina, revealing Lucy's strategies for burying unwanted memory and emotion within appraisals of the lives of others. The nineteenth-century reading audience, coming to *Villette* in the context of the popularity of such works of reminiscence as Tennyson's *In Memoriam* (1850) and Wordsworth's *The Prelude* (1850), would likely have been surprised by this fictional autobiography's departure not only from the attempted reconstruction of key events but also from explicit exposure of the intricate problems involved in remembering a life. Rather than approaching these challenges as points of textual interest or opportunities for spiritual growth, Lucy's recollections are driven by silent tactics for avoiding the need to confront the existence of a problematic past.

That Lucy is orphaned very early in life is clear. Lucy's feelings about her lost relatives – in fact, any details about her origins – are distinctly absent from the text. It is not even particularly clear how they died. At first glance it seems they have been lost in a storm at sea, but Lucy's shifting metaphors leave room for doubt. Lucy figures herself not only as passenger or crewmember on her family's ship through the waters of life but even steersman or the actual ship, and therefore wreck, itself. At the heart of her jumbled imagery is the panic-stricken sensation associated with, and transferable to, other kinds of wreck – moral, emotional, social – which might have blighted her family:

> I too well remember a time – a long time, of cold, of danger, of contention. To this hour, when I have the nightmare, it repeats the rush and saltness of briny waves in my throat, and their icy pressure on my lungs ... For many days neither sun nor stars appeared ... all hope that we should be saved was taken away.[11]

If Lucy 'too well' remembers her past, it is a sense of destructive intensity, rather than any specificity of detail, which leaves its imprint on her narrative and, it appears, her conscious mind. Even the briny nightmare which she claims here as repeating violently is rarely mentioned again, lost in the swash of the workings of Lucy's memory as she searches for a way to express the inexpressible.

Brontë was well aware of the difficulty of achieving genuine expression of unwieldy and complex heightened emotion, of finding a means in language to represent pain and mourning experienced on such a scale that they are felt to be almost inexpressible. Writing to Elizabeth Gaskell in 1850, Brontë provides an assessment of Tennyson's recently published grief-epic, *In Memoriam*, which goes some way towards explaining the artistic choices behind *Villette*'s narrative fits and starts and jagged edges. Speaking in the context of her own recent bereavements, she writes of closing *In Memoriam* when 'I had got about half-way':

> It is beautiful; it is mournful; it is monotonous. Many of the feelings expressed bear, in their utterance, the stamp of Truth, yet if Arthur Hallam had been somewhat nearer Alfred Tennyson – his brother instead of his friend – I should have distrusted this rhymed and measured and printed monument of grief. What change the lapse of years may work – I do not know – but it seems to me that bitter sorrow, while recent, does not flow out in verse.[12]

That which is rhymed and measured, offering itself for readerly admiration as aesthetically pleasing elegy, gives rise to Brontë's misgivings regarding its authenticity. Edward Young's *Night-Thoughts on Life, Death, and Immortality*, an earlier example of such an elegant monument, with which Brontë is also likely to have been familiar,[13] seeks piously to shape the loss of family into 'Inestimable Gain!' Young posits '*Grief!*' as a necessary 'school', where '*Wisdom* smiles, when humbled Mortals weep. / When *Sorrow* wounds the Breast', but there is no such reversal of traumatic loss for Lucy in *Villette*, where it remains unclear whether she has either ability or inclination to 'raise a Tax on my Calamity, / And reap rich Compensation for my Pain'.[14] In fact, despite the beauty of its contours, Tennyson's poem was not insincere, as Brontë's appraisal might suggest. Consuming years of revision, *In Memoriam* ultimately manages to express the merest 'outline' of the poet's 'unquiet' despair.[15] Contained somewhere in the shrouded, impenetrable heart of the poem's monumental form, enduring sorrow remains frustratingly beyond precise verbal reach, and yet stands powerfully in need of expression. Words are but a flimsy outermost layer; narcotics to numb the pain; a 'sad mechanic exercise':

> I sometimes hold it half a sin
> To put in words the grief I feel;
> For words, like Nature, half reveal
> And half conceal the Soul within.[16]

What 'change the lapse of years may work' on her own fresh experience of loss, Brontë in 1850 and perhaps 1853 could 'not know'; Lucy Snowe's 'bitter sorrow', hardly dulled after the softening influence of decades, neither flows out in verse nor prose, but emerges haltingly, and incomplete. Lucy's obsessive self-analysis is repetitive, painfully exacting, yet hardly penetrating. Brontë demonstrates how, by dwelling intensively on present manifestations of psychic discord without sounding their experiential depths, the effects of arrested memory might be exacerbated.

The narrative currents of *Villette*, rather than the narrator's explicit analysis, reveal how the unspoken traumatic past exerts an undeniable stranglehold on the present and future. Pervading the entire novel, this dynamic is clearly established in the mental shifts and ebbs occurring even as Lucy sets sail for the new horizon of Labassecour. With 'nothing to lose', and claiming a guiding bravery emanating from those vague 'terrors' which have 'inured' her to suffering,[17] Lucy attempts to transform her past into a foreign country from which total departure might be possible. Upon landing, however, and within the space of a single paragraph, Lucy's hopeful sense of possessing 'something of the artist's faculty of making the most' of new pleasures diminishes until, observing the vista, she sees only 'slimy' canals and monotonous 'gray'. Attempting to replace the failed vision with poetic rapture (where 'fancy' buds 'fresh' amidst 'deadening influences'), she yet recoils from momentary optimism, describing the process by which any 'feelings' of 'sunshine' she might entertain are perpetually 'kept in check by the secret but ceaseless consciousness of anxiety lying in wait on enjoyment, like a tiger crouched in a jungle'.[18]

Here Brontë figures unquiet memory as a 'beast of prey' at once constantly present yet not able clearly to be seen – let alone identified – by her suffering narrator. That anxiety which Lucy personifies and externalizes as tiger-like, breathing threats into her ear, springs from the trauma lodged within her own panting heart and mental 'lair'.[19] If the jungle of her memory is overgrown, providing cover for stalking unease, it is also boundless, tied to self as well as place. Her 'unsupported mind' drifts with her to Villette,[20] poised to seek anchor in patterns of avoidance, ill health and adversity rather than revelation, change and calm.

Brontë's interest in the mental disjunctions, clashes and disorderings brought about by traumatic memory is evident in the way Lucy's story unfolds, bereft in parts of a strong sense of chronological time and often obscuring the most immediate relations between persons and things. When Lucy arrives in Villette, she is assisted by a man whom she describes as a stranger, and yet trusts infinitely. At the end of Chapter 10, reflecting upon Madame Beck's physician, she registers something 'new' about his appearance with 'the force of surprise, and also of conviction',[21] yet it is many chapters later that Lucy chooses to reveal to the reader that Dr John is not only the man who assisted her upon her arrival but also the John Graham Bretton of her childhood fixation. When Lucy breaks in upon Madame Beck's guests, having encountered the nun's 'ghost', she further embeds John in the narrative as an unidentified man among the party: somewhat odd, given that he has been uppermost in her thoughts, his written words bringing bliss to her senses only moments before. Lucy's familiarity with contemporary scientific terminology explodes into the novel at this point, where the 'unfortunate' curse of obsession she had sought to attribute to Paulina's youthful affection now describes her own distress at losing John's letter, as she refers to herself in the third person clinical view as 'the grovelling, groping, monomaniac'.[22] Like the childhood losses which she refuses or is simply unable to recount, despite their emergence in other ways, Dr John's importance in Lucy's world is communicated by Brontë through the bizarre patterns of his displacement from the text and his various identities within it. The picture, that is to say, is fragmented, and it records the narrator's passage beyond the safe harbours of mental health and equanimity.

The powerfully defensive, if 'paranoid',[23] aspects of Lucy's evasions have been much noted. Of fresh interest here is how obsession, particularly erotic obsession – seemingly a heightened focus of *both* memory and present thought on one object, as explored in the works of Jean Étienne Esquirol and James Cowles Prichard – becomes, in Brontë's text, tightly bound in the narrator's traumatic blocking on an apparently unconscious level, as well as involving the act of intentional forgetting.[24] Brontë develops the particular example of Dr John, and Lucy's interactive processes of yearning and repression, in such a way as to demonstrate the manner in which Lucy's wider willed mnemonic misplacements come to influence, enter into an exchange with, and even overtake, her unconscious (or unwilled) traumatic blanks. Withholding recognition, she reports, 'suited my habits of thought' and 'assimilated with my system of feeling',[25] but it is significant that, in choosing to defer communication of knowledge not only from John but also from the reader, Lucy almost manages to efface it from the text of her life. The internal battle which Lucy represents as occurring between Reason and Feeling when composing variant letters to John embodies a conflict between adopting personal blankness (the erasure of subjective truth by false text or even a tabula rasa) and giving free rein to a desire which (never definitively transcribed or admitted in the text) would speak of continuing links with the past. Envisaging 'life' as a 'war', which 'it seemed my destiny to conduct ... single-handed',[26] the shell-shocked narrator resolves that she will not be laid siege to by memory. In covering herself 'with a cloud' that could not be 'seen through',[27] Brontë shows, Lucy's tactical resistance to avowals of identity obscures her not only from the view (and potential emotional ambush) of others, but also from her own perceptive ability.

Seeking to diminish her capacity for painful recollection, the narrator actively narrows what nineteenth-century writers on memory such as James Douglas and Thomas Brown referred to as the illuminated space of conscious awareness, pointing the searchlight of genuine inquiry steadfastly outwards.[28] While Lucy's 'ray of special illumination' enables insight into others, it 'cast[s] light no farther'.[29] Insofar as they prevent misjudgement by other characters, Lucy's scenes of non-recognition may be seen as critically disruptive, a metatextual challenge from Brontë regarding the ethics of the reading position. Much as it 'works on us by kinds of shock',[30] however, the novel is not simply a proto-modernist experiment with narrative convention. I argue that Lucy's audible narrative silences and subversions of chronology are presented by Brontë as dysfunctional rather than fortifying – elected as a form of attempted empowerment, but having ultimately the obverse effect.

Recounting her strategy for dealing with the blinding attraction of John, Brontë's narrator unwittingly reveals the mode of closing off from insight into the past which structures her approach to the desired retrievals of autobiography. She simply does not look, closing her eyes when vision is thrust upon her. Valuing present pain – the very reliability of the ongoing struggle for survival – Lucy enlists memory against itself, superimposing a restricted, representative image upon any other cues or associations which flash before her. Reflection – encompassed both literally (as an image to be looked at) and figuratively (contemplation or thought) in the spy-mirrors of Rue Fossette – is replaced by a much safer, unchanging form of portraiture.

> I'll tell you what I do, Paulina ... *I never see him.* I looked at him twice or thrice about a year ago, before he recognized me, and then I shut my eyes; and if he were to cross their balls twelve times between each day's sunset and sunrise, except from memory, I should hardly know what shape had gone by.[31]

Although Lucy claims to 'value vision', she dreads 'being struck stone blind' by insight into the past.[32]

'Dry Materialist Views' and the Problem of Female Passion: Doubting the Doctor's Verdict

As Janet Gezari has observed, '*Villette* is as alert to what remains invisible, outside the scope of scientific apprehension, as it is to the increased visibility the individual gains by coming under the doctor's eye'.[33] Dr John and Lucy both undermine the potential significance of external impressions and events when assessing her chronic distress, an unfortunate reality pointed up with some irony by Brontë when it emerges that the 'ghost' of the nun is indeed no spectral illusion but, like Lucy herself, a real person 'in disguise'.[34] As such, their mode of analysis forestalls insight into those hallucinations and inner disturbances that do occur as the result of traumatic memory. Brontë's own perceptive insight extends further than the descriptions offered by characters in the text. Their attempts to understand Lucy's intense feelings and disordered states as the symptoms solely of emotional weakness or psychosomatic malady – causes located firmly in the present, and, essentially, viewed as the 'fault' of the sufferer – are shown to prevent recognition of the need for an examination of, or a coming to terms with, her turbulent history.

At mid-century, as an anonymous article on 'The Passions' in Forbes Winslow's *Journal of Psychological Medicine and Mental Pathology* phrased it, a 'woman's whole life' was said to be a 'history of the affections': she 'embarks her whole soul in the traffic of affection; and if shipwrecked, her case is hopeless, for it is a bankruptcy of the heart'.[35] In conjunction with this, we might consider the scientific community's overarching belief in women's greater susceptibility to and diminished powers of control over nervous disturbances, evident in the rationale of Laycock's *A Treatise on the Nervous Diseases of Women*,[36] and elucidated in J. G. Millingen's view that 'the intellectual powers of woman are inferior to those of man'. For Millingen, with rare exceptions, 'woman' possesses 'less of the *volitional*' and more '*emotional* and *instinctive*' power, which 'frequently become the leading springs of action'.[37] The strain of keeping her 'passions' in check,[38] both in indignant response to these views and for fear of being judged in accordance with them, is shown by Brontë to compound Lucy's trauma, and to complicate her efforts at self-representation.

Disputing Dr John's appeal to the 'nervous system' in favour of the term 'low-spirited',[39] and rejecting M. Paul's recourse to the language of courage and of physiognomy, despite employing similar vocabularies herself at other times, Lucy intermittently endorses physiological definition as she attempts to resist the authoritative male gaze. The language and ideas of contemporary physiological theory are brought into a more potent and expansive metaphorical usage, as when Lucy describes 'a feeling' in terms that she thinks Dr John 'will understand': like a heart 'aneurism' having 'pained my mind'.[40] Brontë, through Lucy, 'objects less to the idea of an interrelationship between body and mind', than to the 'rather partial vision of this union'[41] propounded by theories which reduced mind to body, claiming purely physical causes (malfunctioning of the nerves and organs) for mental and psychic disturbances. Nervous maladies were widely perceived within Victorian society as rather physiological than psychological in nature, thought to arise from the literal stretching or exhaustion of nervous fibres.[42] As Janet Oppenheim notes, the 'theoretical merger' of female nervous and reproductive systems supported the assumption 'that biology dominated women's lives', meaning that the 'burden of sexual stereotyping bore down even more heavily' on female nervous sufferers than on their male counterparts.[43]

Lucy is exhorted to speak, but the threat of overmastering interpretation is ever-present. Dr John's 'professional' gaze triumphs over her experiential knowledge, which he half expects she will furtively 'conceal'.[44] He is merely 'curious', his intention to 'look' in the capacity of objective clinician producing a detachment that Lucy finds disarming. Her inability to speak calls to mind physician and asylum manager John Conolly's complaint regarding the dangerously open boundaries between (and professional ignorance regarding) forms of temporary derangement, such as Lucy's presumed spectral illusions, and 'incurable' madness worthy of incarceration.[45] The interchangeable use of these terms left the patient in a position of particular vulnerability, which Brontë reflects in Lucy's fear of incriminating speech and her recourse to the protective armour of legal terminology at the moment when medical discourse seems poised only to undermine her claims to accuracy and sanity: 'I never will tell exactly what I saw ... unless some one else sees it too, and then I will give corroborative testimony; but otherwise, I shall be discredited and accused of dreaming'.[46]

Struggling to moderate her responses to emotion and sensation in accordance with a masculinist nineteenth-century philosophy of self-control, Lucy is entranced by the enlivening possibilities of expression when she witnesses Vashti's theatre performance. This enables her recognition of the simplistic nature of Graham's 'branding judgment' in artistic and other arenas.[47] With his 'dry, materialist views', Lucy's diagnostician held 'no communion' with any of the elements of experience and expression that 'belonged to storm' or were 'wild and intense'.[48] These are the very attributes over which (as abundant emotions) Lucy heavy-handedly claims mastery but which (as images of selfhood) form the core of her traumatic experience, and describe the effect of her psychic burials upon her body and mind.

In the doctor's very assurance that he will read in her eye, cheek and unsteady hand the visible manifestations of hidden disturbance lurks what is, for Lucy, the clearest indication that his opinion will inevitably be deficient. Her physician may be 'generous', but he lacks 'perception' and 'intuition'.[49] Unwilling to speak for fear of misinterpretation and stigma; unable to be read by Dr John with depth or precision, Lucy must take her own sage advice and brace herself for diagnostic 'disappointment'.[50]

In the I of the Storm (or, 'Happiness is Not a Potato')

As Henry Holland realized in his *Medical Notes and Reflections*, the challenge of finding words which will adequately portray the workings of the mind and memory, in sickness and in health, has 'perplexed reasoning men in every age'.[51] Recoiling against Dr John's verdict in 'secret horror', Lucy seems verbally to acquiesce: 'Is there no cure? – no preventive?'[52] Told to 'cultivate happiness', she manages only a brief response, turning the directive against her interlocutor. Her inner thoughts, however, express firmer opposition, catching up in their condemnatory sweep similar 'advice' contained in numerous nineteenth-century treatises. Dr John's confounding truism that 'a cheerful mind' is the 'preventive' of 'long-continued mental conflict' provides little comfort. Thinks Lucy, 'No mockery in this world ever sounds to me so hollow as that of being told to *cultivate* happiness ... Happiness is not a potato' to be tended so much as 'a divine dew' bestowed upon the soul from 'Paradise'.[53]

If happiness is a 'divine dew', then mental torment is, in Lucy's range of representation, closely aligned with fever and storm: and it is to the narrator's attempts to picture unease through disease, linking atmospheric conditions and the threat of contagion with emotional instability, that I shall now turn.

When the elderly Lucy Snowe records her youthful experience of playing nursemaid, confined behind 'the steam-dimmed lattice of [the] sick-chamber', she betrays an awareness of the effect of this shared air in terms of a crossover between physical and emotional contagion: 'two hot, close rooms thus became my world', and 'all within me became narrowed to my lot'.[54] Breathing the exhalations of the invalid, this most evasive of narrators may certainly hold her own peculiar reasons for embracing a closed world view, but nonetheless demonstrates awareness of the dangers of an infected, claustrophobic atmosphere, where physical stasis curtails, or even contaminates, mental life: 'I forgot that there were fields, woods, rivers, seas, an everchanging sky ... I demanded no walks in the fresh air'. While not – yet – sharing the illness of fever or age, she emulates their symptom of torpor, content to 'crawl ... on' with no more 'appetite' (of any kind) than her charge.[55]

In this concise yet crucial early episode, Brontë forcefully suggests that the invalid's passing leaves Lucy the 'possessor', in addition to fifteen pounds, of a potentially invaluable insight into traumatic testimony. Miss Marchmont gives Lucy 'the originality of her character to study',[56] uttering a final prose ode to Memory which makes clear not only the impossibility of escaping either life's agonies or the memory of their occurrence, but also the potential for transcendence available only through the experience of painful recollection. The extent to which Miss Marchmont's singular flashback guides the narrator's own responses to past and future trauma is, however, like so much else of vital importance in Lucy's history, left unacknowledged. At the time, as in retrospect, Lucy 'had no words' to describe her own reaction to Miss Marchmont's long-delayed revisiting of the death of her betrothed. Even at the conclusion of her own life narrative, following another major loss similar to that sustained by Miss Marchmont, *Villette* leaves open the possibility that Lucy moves on '[s]till all [in] inward darkness'.[57]

During that early darkness of night and soul, what Lucy *does* explicitly outline is a sensorially rich theory of miasma, of bad or 'tormented' air. Her ideas will gain resonance in the later scenes of nightmare and contagion during the long vacation, and the passage is worth quoting in full:

> One February night – I remember it well – there came a voice near Miss Marchmont's house, heard by every inmate, but translated, perhaps, only by one. After a calm winter, storms were ushering in the spring. I had put Miss Marchmont to bed; I sat at the fireside sewing. The wind was wailing at the windows: it had wailed all day; but, as night deepened, it took a new tone – an accent keen, piercing, almost articulate to the ear; a plaint, piteous and disconsolate to the nerves, trilled in every gust.

> 'Oh, hush! hush!' I said in my disturbed mind, dropping my work, and making a vain effort to stop my ears against that subtle, searching cry. I had heard that very voice ere this, and compulsory observation had forced on me a theory as to what it boded. Three times in the course of my life, events had taught me that these strange accents in the storm – this restless, hopeless cry – denote a coming state of the atmosphere unpropitious to life. Epidemic diseases, I believed, were often heralded by a gasping, sobbing, tormented, long-lamenting east wind. Hence, I inferred, arose the legend of the Banshee. I fancied, too, I had noticed – but was not philosopher enough to know whether there was any connection between the circumstances – that we often at the same time hear of disturbed volcanic action in distant parts of the world; of rivers suddenly rushing above their banks; and of strange high tides flowing furiously in on low sea-coasts. 'Our globe', I had said to myself, 'seems at such periods torn and disordered; the feeble amongst us wither in her distempered breath, rushing hot from steaming volcanoes'.[58]

Though disavowing possession of insight into the connections between epidemic diseases, banshee winds, volcanic action and tidal disturbance, Brontë's narrator yet advances a sense of the scale of connection, or spread – where the whole globe seems torn by unease, if not disease-related strife – and isolates a concern common among writers of medical texts and advice literature: that it is the 'feeble amongst us' who 'wither', or succumb, under pressure of unexpected external changes in weather and air-freshness. It is as if the feeble take on their fevers directly from the air rushing hot from distant steaming volcanoes.

Brontë's representation of extreme physiologic sympathy brings into play a kind of global environmental development of the late eighteenth-century cult of sensibility. It takes up, on a large scale, Lucy Snowe's later concern with the invisible 'chords of sympathy' between individuals, and imagines the prediction and transmission of disease along similar lines, with the sympathy here between the susceptible individual and the distempered earth. Intriguingly, Brontë presents Lucy's ideas about global distemper not only in order to develop important connections between sympathy, health and suffering but also to suggest ways in which Lucy's self-analysis in autobiographical writing will continually miss the mark. For Brontë, the storms that recur throughout *Villette* presage not only fever and disease but, vitally, the onset of traumatic memory. If the keening voice of the wind, 'heard by every inmate' of Miss Marchmont's house, but 'translated, perhaps, only by one', is understood by Lucy as the language of death, its screams awaken that 'quick' of her nature – memory – which she has 'studiously' held 'in catalepsy and a dead trance'.[59] Tumultuous weather stirs 'a craving cry I could not satisfy':[60] the cry for release which will only be enabled by remembrance. Lucy strives hopelessly to 'stop' her ears 'against that subtle, searching cry',[61] which she links with the onset of three former instances of unspecified destruction, and attempts rationally to place the association amidst global events. Her movement from talk of epidemics and 'volcanic action' to – closer to the central traumatic metaphor – 'strange high tides' gives rise to the question whether it was such a storm as this that occurred immediately prior to the loss of her family during childhood – resulting in both its figurative encasement in terms of shipwreck, and her current reaction. If wild weather – and the eerie after-storm 'dead calm' – are harbingers of death, it is not the death of multitudes but of known individuals: a closer and perhaps more difficult reality to recount.

For eighteenth-century physician and Professor of the Theory of Medicine at the University of Edinburgh, Robert Whytt,

> there is a remarkable sympathy, by means of the nerves, between the various parts of the body; and now it appears that there is a still more wonderful sympathy between the nervous systems of different persons whence various motions and morbid symptoms are often transferred, from one to another, without any corporeal contact or infection.[62]

Thomas John Graham also writes of the role of sympathy in producing fever, pointing towards the potential for sympathy both between organs and between people:

> The chief predisposing cause is debility, however induced; but the grand exciting cause is marsh miasma, or the effluvia arising from stagnant water, or marshy ground, impregnated with vegetable matter in a state of putrefactive decomposition. Dampness, and the night air, are particularly favourable to the full operation of marsh miasma. Ague [or fever] does arise, however, from other causes than marsh effluvia; and it may be produced by sympathy, or [by] irritation in the stomach and intestines.[63]

Bereft of the company of others over the long vacation, and forced to conclude that *imagined* chords of sympathy with others are precisely that, Lucy Snowe's thoughts are left to fold in upon themselves – not unlike a miasmic breeding ground, her unexamined past in 'a state of putrefactive decomposition' that becomes, at last, impossible to ignore.

Robert Burton's *Anatomy of Melancholy*, written in 1621 and continually revised and corrected until the posthumous sixth edition of 1651, was a popular nineteenth-century reference. The Brontës owned an abridged edition of 1827, and a two-volume version was available at the Keighley Mechanics' Institute Library. In its unabridged form, the work ends with a 'short precept' for the reader seeking to 'tenderest thine owne welfare', 'ease his afflicted minde, relieve his wounded soule, and take him out of the jawes of hell it selfe': '*Be not solitary, be not idle*'.[64] This sentiment is both echoed and directly quoted in numerous early- to mid-nineteenth-century writings on disorders affecting the mind, outweighing Romantic notions of solitude as, primarily, providing a reflective mental space. Samuel Taylor Coleridge's lime-tree bower, for example, transmogrifies from prison to protective meditative enclosure once its potential and meaning are properly comprehended – an awareness reached only through the process of reflection enforced by the seeming incarceration, suggesting the strong Romantic link between solitude and the positive expansion of consciousness.[65] Numerous Victorian writers on the mind in phases of illness recommend 'separation' from family and a change of scene, to break the chain 'of morbid ideas' attendant upon the initial experience of unrest.[66] A significant number, however, insist that for those suffering permanent or temporary mental derangement, the perils of solitariness outweigh the benefits. While James Cowles Prichard writes that '[q]uiet seclusion' is beneficial for patients exhibiting 'wildness of conduct', he considers that, when treating individuals with a 'habitual fondness of solitude', it is of utmost importance that this 'disposition should be as much as possible counteracted'.[67] Lucy perpetually seeks the 'stillness' of her own company, drawn by 'the very gloom' and cover of the attic and garden after dusk.[68] By choice and by circumstance, her patterns of habitation, hence mind and narrative, share an overarching atmosphere of constriction and claustrophobia.

Brontë's novel explores a mid-nineteenth-century preoccupation with evaluating the extent to which, in John Reid's words, the 'society in the centre of which a person is placed, may be regarded as the atmosphere of his mind'.[69] This engagement, encompassing concerns with urban overcrowding and the risk of contagion, centred on the need for meaningful structures of community. Making reference to Burton's *Anatomy of Melancholy*, Reid proposed that it is 'not so much from a stagnation of air, as from the want of a free circulation and ventilation ... of thought, that some of those diseases which we are the least able to bear, are most apt to originate'.[70] Lucy's mind suffocates when, focused upon the single conscious idea of her painful loneliness, thought begins to stagnate, threatening annihilation. Her greatest fear is that of complete erasure by being literally unremembered. Seclusion becomes exclusion becomes extinguishment from others' living memory, a fate equal to literal death: 'It kills me to be forgotten'.[71] Reid, on 'Solitude', concurs: the 'lamp of life burns to waste in the sepulchre of solitude'.[72]

Lucy is able to summarize the first monotonous month of the vacation as 'long, black, heavy',[73] like a mental storm cloud (a later life-chapter, following the 'Sunshine' of Pauline and Graham's marriage, is simply entitled 'Cloud'). Brontë's narrator is shown to experience to some degree what Reid refers to as 'the contagious quality of mental depression'[74] – if the servant Goton in 'far distant attic' is hardly registered, the 'mopping and mowing' of the disabled student or crétin whom Lucy tends magnifies her repulsion at her own 'warped' mind, with its mnemonic 'wasting and wearing'.[75] Despite its internal temporal derangements (the experience of the crétin described, after her removal; the hint of storm and of fever pervading the passage, before the breaking of either), this ordeal remains readily available to conscious recall for the older Lucy, who cannot 'ever forget it'.[76] So horrifyingly memorable are those desolate days, because bound up with the return of other memories to which – as to hope – her heart and mind had attempted to draw an 'inhospitable bar to admission'.[77] Like the very solitude she endures, Lucy becomes (as in the opening words of Reid's essay on 'Solitude', taken from the *Art of Health*) the 'sad nurse of care' to 'sickly musing' and the 'dim-eyed fiend, / Sour Melancholy', which 'night and day provokes / Her own eternal wound'.[78] In Brontë's estimation, as in Reid's, it is essential that a person 'carry into [solitude] a mind unincumbered with painful remembrances, and unwounded by the infliction of any great calamity'.[79]

Lucy's autobiographical testimony makes it *appear* that she has managed to evade the mental outworkings of trauma in nightmare until the final two weeks of isolation. Closer analysis reveals this to be another dimension in which Brontë explores the effacement of memory as a form of silencing control that infects the wider life narrative. Dream, nightmare, and even the blank interstices of sleep function as trigger words or quietly resounding fears regarding the resurgence of past reality in the text. The admitted recurrence of Lucy's choking salty nightmare – said to 'repeat' upon her even '[t]o this hour' of writing – combines strangely with the infrequency of its mention, suggestively seeping into hollow textual spaces. Brontë devises a narrator concerned with recounting not the shackles of memory but the spirit's shaking of 'its always-fettered wings half loose',[80] a narrator who will ignore bad dreams, like bad air or distempered thought, where possible – though their constant presence in her life will be indicated in other ways, particularly through this evident reliance on narratorial elision. It is in pointedly general and detached language that Lucy observes that night is 'an unkindly time' for 'the solitary': 'strange starts and struggles harass his couch'.[81] Brontë, having Lucy assume the masculine pronoun, embeds in her narrator's vivid description the intensity of her efforts to distance herself from uncomfortable reality, pitying some anonymous 'Poor wretch!' rather than directly claiming his story as her own.

The nightmare that occurs during the long vacation coincides with actual 'equinoctial' storms,[82] the onset of which equates also with Lucy's descent into physical illness, and thus its representation can hardly be avoided. Her sense of time becomes 'bewildered' under the force of the hurricane: for 'nine dark and wet days ... the Hours rushed on all turbulent, deaf, dishevelled'.[83] Past, present and future, the very seasons, are caught up in the temporal whirlpool, and their interrelationship can no longer be obtrusively obscured by mind or by narrative. Febrility, combined with the external storm (which, here as elsewhere, is never a 'casual' circumstance but a 'cry' laced with warning),[84] reawakens the sleeping past in the mind of the wakeful narrator.

Henry Holland and George Man Burrows both speculate about the influence of weather in relation to disease. For Holland, thunder and even strong winds cause electrical changes in the atmosphere which may affect the 'blood and nervous system', causing sensations 'oppressive and singular'.[85] In Burrows's view, nervous sufferers are 'extremely susceptible of atmospheric changes'.[86] Brontë opens up for the reader's analysis Lucy's statement that 'I do not know why that change in the atmosphere made a cruel impression on me'.[87] Electrifying Lucy's mental atmosphere, the 'beating rain' breaks down the barriers between life and metaphor, bringing the unassimilated past like a lightning bolt into the present. Prompting associative memory, the storm reminds the reader, as it must Lucy, of the events underlying her assumption of the imagery of watery destruction. Amidst insomnia and fitful exhaustion, Sleep comes but once: she comes 'in anger', provoking Lucy's 'avenging dream',[88] or traumatic flashback.

As Janis Caldwell observes in her discussion of Mary Shelley's *Frankenstein*, 'the theory of physiologic sympathy ... posits fragile bodies, susceptible to contagion and collapse. Under this model, social sympathy is safe only for people of nearly identical psychological and somatic constitutions.'[89] This raises the question of the effect of Lucy's narrative upon the reader – as the crétin's physical 'mopping and mowing' calls forth Lucy's mental 'wasting and wearing', does the whole create a textual atmosphere 'unpropitious' if not to life then to readerly enjoyment? Harriet Martineau and Matthew Arnold, both of whom reviewed the novel's intensity of purpose and 'atmosphere of [unremitting] pain' unfavourably, would almost certainly agree.[90] For George Eliot's partner, scientist George Henry Lewes, on the other hand, *Villette*'s pathological cry 'issues an influence of truth as healthful as the mountain breeze'.[91] The healthful influence seen by Lewes in Brontë's sensitive delineation of states of illness may be precisely the narrative's call for a widening conception of the mnemonic, traumatic causes of mental, emotional and physical suffering.

Having found her ideal partner and listening audience in one; 'the next day – he sailed'.[92] The storm of Lucy's mind returns to haunt her as a horrifying reality unfolds. While her unnamed, unnumbered kinsfolk were lost in what Lucy viewed in vague metaphorical terms as the 'wreck' following years traversing troubled waters, Monsieur Paul becomes the literal victim of shipwreck and drowning, though this is never directly admitted in the text. Instead, the Banshee winds return as harbinger of death:

> I know some signs of the sky; I have noted them since childhood. God, watch that sail! Oh! Guard it!
>
> The wind shifts to the west. Peace, peace, Banshee – 'keening' at every window! It will rise – it will swell – it shrieks out long: wander as I may through the house this night, I cannot lull the blast ...
>
> The storm roared frenzied for seven days ... it did not lull till the deeps had gorged their full of sustenance. Not till the destroying angel of tempest had achieved his perfect work, would he fold the wings whose waft was thunder – the tremor of whose plumes was storm.[93]

Lucy employs the pretence of concern for the overtaxed or disappointed readerly imagination, covering her own grief with the instruction here to 'pause: pause at once', and be silent, 'there is enough said'. In seeking benevolently to 'trouble no quiet, kind heart; leave sunny imaginations hope',[94] Brontë's narrator once again stoppers up the turmoil inside her own unquiet mind, concealing beneath a reticent aesthetic response to death the immovability of a mind perhaps this time irrevocably stunned. Lucy's narrative has shown that the replacement of expressed grief and resultant emotional growth by an 'amiable conjecture' of false happiness will wreak monumental and enduring 'harm',[95] despite deliberate protestation to the contrary. This signals the danger encased in the words 'there is enough said'. There has not been enough said, at all. Leaving readers who so choose to 'picture union and a happy succeeding life' – despite the mortal 'hush' and disturbingly dark sunlight that separates herself, fragmented into a 'thousand weepers', from the sound of her beloved's voice – the white-haired Lucy is, even now, years after this second traumatic fatality, left stranded and alone in the absolute blank of aftermath and mnemonic incapacity. Unable to name her loss, Brontë's narrator cannot even seek comfort in the anticipated empathy of readers, drawing back from full autobiographical disclosure, and stopped short by the pain of memory 'dim as a wheel fast spun'.[96]

In *Villette*, the mid-nineteenth-century fascination with stagnation of air and suffocation of mind coincide, bringing together mnemonic disruptions of body and mind to develop a nineteenth-century vision of trauma, or mental shock, that encompasses notions of storm, 'tormented' winds, and local and global atmospheres 'unpropitious to life'. The 'compulsory observation' of *Villette*'s narrator Lucy Snowe is structured by Brontë in such a way as to suggest that, although only certain receptive minds might be attuned to the emergent 'theory' of psychic trauma, it will not be solely the 'feeble' in Victorian society who are disposed physically to 'wither' under the pressures of mnemonic disruption. Lucy's representation breaks free from the diagnostic categories within which much female experience was delimited and contained. The shifting choice and use of scientific terms employed in her ongoing attempt at self-description demonstrates the need for modes of insight that allow for 'communion' between what Lucy sees as 'dry materialist views' and those elements of experience and expression that 'belonged to storm' or were 'wild and intense' (without denoting a lesser intellect, or total immersion in 'passion' over reason, as Millingen and other mid-nineteenth-century writers would suggest). In large part, for Brontë, the task of picturing women's mental unease is precisely that of picturing the conditions of certain states of mind (in stagnation and distemper) that have causes quite distinct from those prevailing gendered constructs that might most limit understanding. For, while the frame within which Lucy's self-portrait rests is largely determined along gendered lines in terms of social opportunities for women, her reactions to wider circumstances of catastrophic loss are drawn in markedly broader, human terms. In Brontë's final novel, traumatic suffering is shown to result from an overwhelming external shock or blow – not from pre-existing hysteria, madness or anxiety. Mnemonic disturbance is shown to proceed, between and primarily within individuals, in patterns echoing storm and contagion, and with startling miasmic textual effects: 'Indeed', as Lucy Snowe remarks, 'there was no way to keep well under the circumstances'.[97]

5 THE ICONOGRAPHY OF ANOREXIA NERVOSA IN THE LONG NINETEENTH CENTURY

Susannah Wilson

In 2010 the French model and actress Isabelle Caro died from complications arising as a result of her fifteen-year struggle with anorexia nervosa. Three years prior to her death, as a statement against the fashion industry's promotion of excessive thinness, Caro's naked image was displayed on billboards in Italy to coincide with Milan Fashion Week, carrying the message 'No Anorexia'. Caro claimed that she weighed around 27 kg (59lb) at the time.[1] Previously, in 2006–7 three South American models in their early twenties had starved themselves to death: the Brazilian Ana Carolina Reston and sisters Eliana and Luisel Ramos from Uruguay, resulting in widespread criticism of the use of 'size 0' models and placing the issue of the visibility of anorexia firmly on the public agenda.

Regrettably, Caro is more famous for her anorexia than for her acting or modelling career, which reveals something of the extent of public fascination with this disease. Anorexia is marked by a visibility shared by few other illnesses, with only severe skin disorders and facial disfigurements being as visually striking. Its presence in cultural imagery therefore holds a peculiar significance, a unique ability to make an arresting statement about how women inhabit their bodies. Today, the iconography of the disease exists predominantly in the domain of popular culture: a Google search will produce millions of images of emaciated young women, for the most part published in unofficial blogs and controversial pro-anorexia ('pro-Ana') forums. Conversely, however, contemporary mainstream medical and psychiatric journals never reproduce photographs of anorexic women.[2]

But this has not always been the case. During the period 1873–1914, there was a surge of interest in an illness found among young girls from the privileged classes, characterized by the refusal of food and extreme emaciation, and which seemed distinct from organic wasting illnesses such as chlorosis and tuberculosis. This interest was generated by the simultaneous naming of the disease as *anorexia nervosa* by the eminent Victorian physician Sir William Gull and *ano-*

rexie hystérique by Charles Lasègue, an influential French psychiatrist based at La Pitié hospital in Paris, in the 1870s.[3] A number of publications that followed in their wake were illustrated with graphic clinical portraits of its victims.

Although the problem of self-starvation has been observed since at least the medieval era, the date of 1873 is significant in terms of the wider recognition of the disorder that occurred following Lasègue's and Gull's naming of the disease. Joan Jacobs Brumberg has made a compelling case for viewing the nineteenth century as the historical period that marked the emergence of anorexia nervosa as a *modern* phenomenon: it was not considered by doctors to be a disease requiring medical treatment before this date, and it began to be interpreted as a cultural problem in the twentieth century. Brumberg's wide-ranging history includes some discussion of Gull's clinical portraits,[4] and the present essay adds a new level of detail to the historical study of anorexia by considering Gull's anorectics alongside a number of contemporary cases which have not previously been discussed in the secondary literature. Whilst Lasègue did not include pictures in his famous paper, illustrated cases of anorexia were published by other authors in prestigious journals such as the *Lancet* and the *Nouvelle Iconographie de la Salpêtrière*, as well as in individual medical treatises and less prominent journals, such as the *Medical Press and Circular*. The cases singled out for commentary in this essay are interpreted in the light of broader theoretical perspectives on the iconography of disease, and the insights offered by psychoanalytical approaches to anorexia and to the theory of the 'gaze'.[5]

In the late nineteenth and early twentieth centuries, clinical portraits were often used in the optimistic hope of demonstrating the efficacy of treatment.[6] Later, the practice of photographing anorectics declined as an awareness of the intractability of the disease grew. Whilst many of these early, illustrated publications are well known to historians, little critical attention has been paid to the function of the images they contain. Focusing on fifteen clinical portraits, this essay argues that the visibility of anorexia generates a profoundly ambivalent response to the emaciated female body. Whilst it fascinates us, it also disrupts gender norms, institutional hierarchies and sacred social rituals. Central to this ambivalent reaction is the question of control, and this essay suggests that the anorexic body – far from being mastered by either patient or doctor – emerges as an uncontrollable and yet highly meaningful entity.

Brumberg convincingly demonstrates that nineteenth-century clinicians, following in the tradition of Lasègue and Gull, did not seek to understand the meaning of anorexia from the perspective of the young women who lived and died in its grip. Freud would be the first to do this: 'Freud posed the important conceptual question that had not been asked before: What does the anorectic's lack of appetite *mean*?'[7] When Freud – who said very little about anorexia – first linked appetite to libido, and Pierre Janet identified the problem of self-loathing in relation to the body, the way was paved for a more nuanced psychodynamic view of anorexia.[8] Neither of these influential clinicians include in their case reports portraits of patients for whom anorexia nervosa was the primary diagnosis, but their insights marked a departure from the nineteenth-century perspectives of Gull and Lasègue, who believed anorexia was a behaviour that needed to be suppressed through moral control, and a movement towards the current clinical emphasis on understanding the meaning of the disease. This ongoing search for meaning helps us retrospectively to interpret these nineteenth-century clinical portraits, which reveal a tension between doctors' resistance to understanding the psychological significance of food refusal, and the patient's resistance to the 'correction' of a deeply meaningful and perversely empowering behaviour. As Richardson has noted elsewhere in this collection, in the context of nineteenth-century hunger strikers, the refusal of food represented a symbolic weapon against an overbearing and unreasonable society for women who lacked control over the medical interventions imposed on them.

The use of illustrated case studies follows in the nineteenth-century tradition of medical portraiture, particularly the iconography of the insane, a theme explored in greater detail in Ford's essay in this volume. Théodore Géricault's portraits of monomaniacs, commissioned by the prominent French alienist Jean-Étienne Georget in the 1820s, reflect the eighteenth-century model of using physiognomy as a means to detect mental diseases. In England, Alexander Morison's *The Physiognomy of Mental Diseases* in 1840 established the same concern to connect physical appearance to mental pathology.[9] Sander Gilman argues that Hugh Diamond's 1856 paper presented to the Royal Society on the use of photography in psychiatry inaugurated a new era in the iconography of mental diseases. Previously, as Gilman demonstrates, clinical portraits had held a moral and cautionary aim, rather than a clear therapeutic one. Diamond, by contrast, followed in the empirical tradition of the French school represented by Pinel – who believed that mental illness could be cured – in viewing the purpose of medical photography as being to record the appearance of patients for study; it was also recommended for therapeutic use as a means of presenting an accurate self-image back to the patient.[10]

Many highly visible diseases – for example, acromegaly, acne and psoriasis – originally photographed in nineteenth-century editions of the *Nouvelle Iconographie* and the *Lancet* are still frequently included in published medical reports today, but anorexia is not among them. Perhaps anorectics were photographed in order to aid recognition of the disease, which is no longer necessary in an age when the image of the anorectic is part of the cultural consciousness. It may be that photography was used, as a new and impressive technology, to add weight to Gull's clinical argument that anorexia was simple to cure. He demonstrates this through the use of pictures of anorexic patients 'before' and 'after' treatment. This stands in marked contrast to the current perception of the disease as difficult to treat and rarely 'cured'. The Diagnostic and Statistical Manual of Mental Disorders (DSM-IV) reports an 'impressive long-term mortality' rate (10–20 per cent) for those hospitalized for anorexia, and that only 30–50 per cent of anorectics will make 'full and complete psychological and physical recoveries'. The reality is a high rate of relapse, with many requiring hospitalization again within a year, and many others developing chronic eating disorders.[11]

Since the early twentieth century anorexia nervosa is also thought to have become more common. Recent experts such as psychiatrist Hilde Bruch and psychoanalyst Susie Orbach assert that since the 1960s anorexia has grown into an epidemic affecting young women, and argue that the disease in its most modern form has only existed since the advent of the mass media in the early to mid-twentieth century.[12] Indeed, weight phobia as part of the diagnostic picture is only indicated in some of the nineteenth-century cases. Today, it is a necessary diagnostic criterion. Orbach argues that the anorexic woman's struggle may be interpreted as a 'metaphor for our age', as 'an expression of a woman's confusion about how much space she may take up in the world'.[13] This epidemiological shift has coincided with a trend in the medical literature towards the suppression of photographs of patients, but also – paradoxically – with an increased fascination with the anorexic body in popular culture.

The most significant historical events cutting across this change are the two world wars. It is frequently suggested that anorexia is rare or non-existent in communities where hunger is a true physical threat, but since there are examples of cases being reported during wartime in Europe this alone cannot explain the disappearance of clinical photographs.[14] In terms of the events of twentieth-century Europe, however, there is great significance in the imagery of emaciation. Since 1945, mass-media images of starving people have often carried connotations of the immense human suffering inflicted on the weak by the strong: the Holocaust; the Balkans conflicts of the 1990s; and the orphans of the Ceausescu régime in Romania, to cite just a few examples. In this context, depicting an act of wilful self-starvation might seem distasteful. But doctors have not shied away from illustrating distressing diseases, so this is unlikely to be the reason why clinicians stopped photographing anorexic patients. Rather, these images disappeared from clinical literature as the fashion for photographing psychiatric patients waned along with the credence of the study of physiognomy in relation to mental disorders.

There is more than a superficial similarity between victims of food shortages and anorectics, despite the state of the latter being apparently self-inflicted. The anorexic woman typically experiences what has been eloquently described by Marilyn Lawrence as a 'control paradox': although her behaviour exerts tyrannical control over both her body and the people around her, she feels perilously out of control. Far from being able to 'pull herself together', she experiences as little agency over her wasting body as a famine victim. Lawrence argues that those treating anorectics pay too little heed to this paradox, and that the focus on weight gain obscures the need to understand the root causes of the weight loss: '[Doctors] see anorexics as women who are exercising too much self-control. They simply don't take account of the intense feelings of being out of control which accompany this. Thus, therapeutic intervention for them is based on breaking the control.'[15]

The problem of control is a central theme in the case studies analysed in this essay. I argue that doctors used clinical portraits in an attempt to show that anorexia can be controlled; what they actually reveal is the limited extent to which it can be. In 1936, Professor John Ryle gave the Schorstein Memorial Lecture on 'Anorexia Nervosa' at the London Hospital, later to be published in the *Lancet*. Ryle viewed anorexia as a 'habit' that needed to be 'corrected', and asserted: 'Parent and daughter must both be allowed to see that the physician has *a complete grasp of the situation*'.[16] Following a page of vignettes of fatal cases of the disease, Ryle's statement of confidence in the authority of the doctor stands out as staggeringly ironic. This need to control reflects a disturbing lack of control, keenly felt by clinicians, that mirrors the anorectic's own dilemma. Clinical portraits, therefore, are an attempt to substantiate the fantasy of control over the disease.

If the anxiety to control wilful self-starvation is so pressing, these case studies with their haunting illustrations confirm Sander Gilman's observations on clinical portraiture that centre on the need to create images of disease onto which healthy people can project their unconscious distress:

> It is the fear of collapse, the sense of dissolution, which contaminates the Western image of all diseases ... We project this fear onto the world in order to localize it and, indeed to domesticate it. For once we locate it, the fear of our own dissolution is removed. Then it is not we who totter on the brink of collapse, but rather the Other ... The construction of the image of the patient is thus always a playing out of this desire for a demarcation between ourselves and the chaos represented in culture by disease.[17]

With these observations in mind, this essay will argue that images of anorectics are subversive of the 'male gaze', the viewpoint via which they are framed. From Hegel's master–slave dialectic, to Sartre's preoccupation with the aggressor–victim relationship between looker and object, and to Foucault's location of medical power in clinical observation, the significance of the 'gaze' has been heavily theorized.[18] Drawing on this long history, film analyst Laura Mulvey in 1975 outlined a concept of the 'male gaze' as the camera reflecting the perspective of heterosexual man and objectifying women, who in film are 'coded for strong visual and erotic impact'.[19] She draws from this the idea that this limited perspective forces women also to adopt the male gaze, for they are constantly aware of being looked at by men. Mulvey draws on Lacanian psychoanalytic theory to theorize this unequal power relationship, and argues that women thus displayed represent the 'Other' to the man's image of himself, evoking the ultimate castration anxiety; what she means by this is that images of women evoke pleasure but also anxiety for men, because 'castrated' women illustrate the threat that hangs over them.[20] In the case of anorectics, this anxiety is embodied in the threat posed by her resistance to medical treatment, by the fact that her behaviour may not be overcome.

The first group of cases studied here present linear narratives of medical 'cure' and control over the rebellious anorexic patient. These cases are optimistic in tone and tend to see treatment as a simple affair, being based on the correction of a behaviour rather than any meaningful psychological transformation in the patient's attitude to food; they are also likely to be illustrated with 'before' and 'after' images of (post-)anorexic patients to illustrate the success of the hospital regime. These cases can be designated as 'scopophilic' in terms of the male gaze, for the subversive anorexic image is overwritten by the pleasant image of recovery which replicates the style of a portrait of a normal young girl. These images also reveal self-awareness on the part of the women pictured (a sense that they know they are being looked at), suggesting their ambivalent adoption of the male gaze. In the second group of case studies, which report either fatal or inconclusive outcomes, the use of illustrations reveals a morbid fascination with the anorexic body, and therefore can be classified as voyeuristic because the focus is on the sick rather than the recovered body (which is not depicted at all in these cases). This voyeurism is most clearly present in the absolute lack, visually speaking, of the patient's point of view through the obscuring of their faces or the fact that they are photographed dead.[21]

The concealing of the face in this second group of cases is also surprising given the historical importance of physiognomy in psychiatric photography. This concealment lends the images a distinctly voyeuristic quality, and the complex erotic charge communicated as a result also links them to the familiar trope of the wasting female heroine in nineteenth-century art and literature: from Flaubert's *Madame Bovary* (1857) to the chlorotic women depicted in Baudelaire's prose poetry (1869); from the consumptive 'Mimi' portrayed in Puccini's opera *La Bohème* (1896) to Lefebvre's painting *La Blanche Ophélie* (1890) and the near-to-death pose shown in Millais's *Ophelia* (1851–2), a paradoxical fascination with lifeless and yet captivating women was widely expressed. The link between these popular images and the voyeuristic fascination with images of anorexic patients will be further drawn in the second section of this essay.[22]

Narratives of Recovery

Each case to be examined in this first section presents a linear account, beginning with an illustration of emaciation and ending with an image of health, which strongly conforms to the scopophilic expectations of the male gaze. It will be argued that the apparent simplicity of this 'cure' masks a deeper anxiety about the power of the disease and its mysterious aetiology. Compared to the second group of studies, the voices of the patients are less present in the narrative but the patient's appearance in the 'before' images is a subversive presence. Just as the control of the appetite might be read as an expression of the patient's voice, her facial expression, posture and gestures communicate with the viewer.[23] Her initial subversion of, and later compliance with, the framing male gaze reveals a level of self-consciousness on the part of the patient about the meaning of her anorexia.[24] It expresses dissatisfaction with conventional gender expectations, but doctors seek only to erase the symptoms of disease. In doing so, they fail to appreciate its profound cultural significance.

Gull's 1874 paper illustrates the cases of Misses A., B. and C. (Figures 5.1, 5.2, 5.3). Forced feeding is enthusiastically recommended by Gull as the way to deal with food refusal, and he confidently asserts: 'the inclination of the patient must be in no way consulted'.[25] The photograph of Miss A. displays illness through facial expressions and gestures as much as through the appearance of thinness; she is pictured with head inclined, wearing a forlorn expression, wide-eyed, passive and with her hair tied back in the typical style of an old maid. In the second, her hair is styled in curls, in the fashion of young women of the time, and falls prettily around her full cheeks; her expression dignified with a hint of a smile. Gull draws the following contrast: 'It will be noticeable that as she recovered she had a much younger look, corresponding indeed to her age, 21; whilst the photographs, taken when she was 17, give her the appearance of being near 30'.[26] Anorexia leads to degeneration and decline, whereas the re-feeding regime has brought about rejuvenation. Gull and others regard anorectics as being unable to inhabit their bodies in an age-appropriate way; his observations echo the way in which anorexic women are commonly compared to both pre-pubescent girls in refusal of adult sexuality, and to post-menopausal women – the French doctor Georges Gasne, for example, within the same sentence describes his sixteen-year-old patient as striking for her 'haggard' and yet 'girlish' appearance.[27] These comparisons are implicitly linked to the amenorrhea symptomatic of the disease.

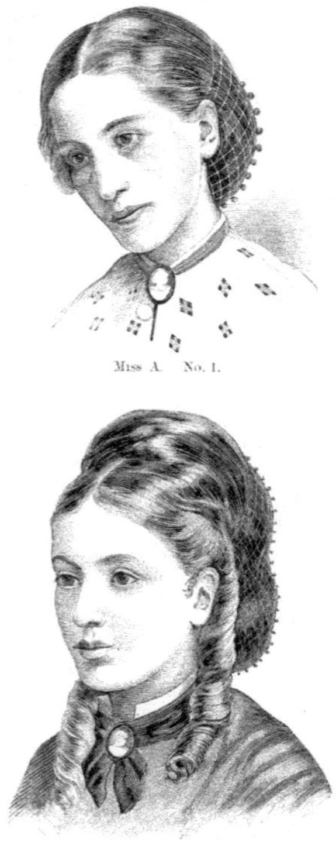

Figure 5.1: Miss A., in W. Gull, 'Anorexia Nervosa,' in T. Dyke Acland (ed.), *A Collection of the Published Writings of William Withey Gull* (1874; London: The New Sydenham Society, 1894), pp. 305–14, on p. 306. Wellcome Library, London.

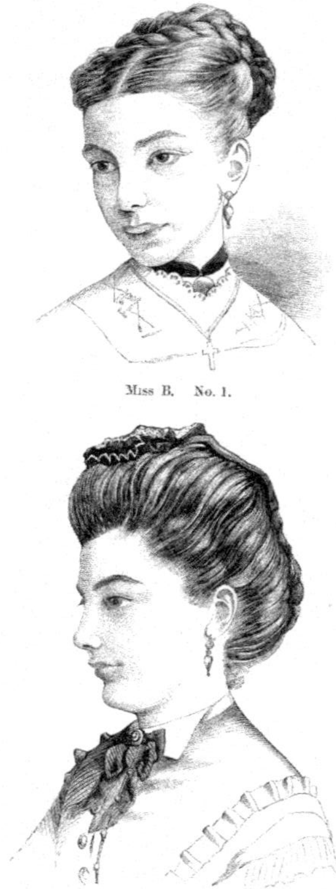

Figure 5.2: Miss B., in Gull, 'Anorexia Nervosa' (1874), p. 308. Wellcome Library, London.

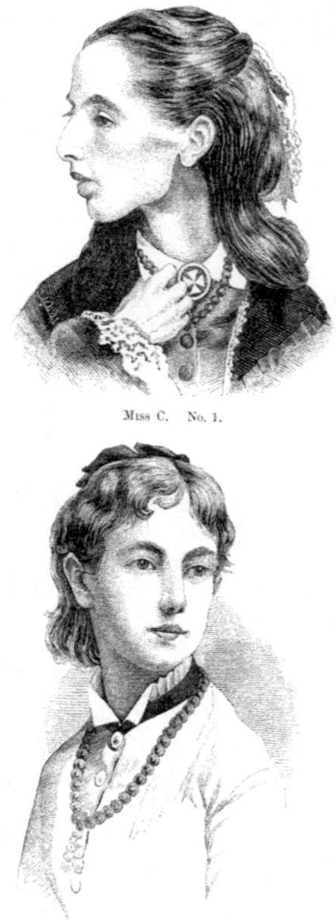

Figure 5.3: Miss C., in Gull, 'Anorexia Nervosa' (1874), p. 310. Wellcome Library, London.

Miss B. does not look obviously different in the 'before' and 'after' images other than a slight plumpness around the chin. By contrast, the third case, Miss C., shows a striking transformation. The report is made up of a series of letters between Gull and a general practitioner colleague, Dr Anderson, who reports her return to being 'plump and rosy as of yore'.[28] Her extreme weight loss is accentuated through the hard line of her jaw, hollow cheeks and stretched skin. She is also depicted turning away, in refusal of the viewer's gaze, repeating the defiance of the previous images. The recovered Miss C. is depicted in half-profile in a movement towards engaging the viewer; her head is held up and her cheeks and lips are visibly fuller.

In his introduction, Gull asserts: 'at present our diagnosis of this affection is negative, so far as determining any positive cause from which it springs'.[29] Gull admits here that he does not really understand what causes the disease, and does not seek to. He does show an early insight, however, in distinguishing anorexia nervosa from emaciation due to organic causes. He argues that the disease is 'due to a morbid mental state', and that his 'wilful patients' need to be placed under strict moral conditions including complete isolation from the family and forced feeding: 'the treatment required is obviously that which is fitted for persons of unsound mind'.[30] Despite Gull's appreciation of the psychological nature of the problem, there is no attempt to see the sufferer's behaviour from her point of view, and there is no evidence of empathy with her distress. These illustrations demonstrate Gull's belief that 'moral control' of the patient is what produces recovery. The plump and smiling faces of his recovered patients show that he had some reason to believe in his methods; what his analysis fails to appreciate is the psychological meaning of the patient's behaviour, which begins to be revealed – albeit in a rather enigmatic way – in the anorexic images.

Thomas Stretch Dowse, a physician at the London Hospital for Epilepsy and Paralysis, published the case of fourteen-year-old A. T. in 1881 (Figure 5.4). She is described as a 'very delicate child' presenting classically anorexic character traits: a 'great obstinacy of disposition' and being prone to 'sullen fits'.[31] Dowse describes in some detail the complex and strained relationships within this girl's family, and claims that treatment only succeeds once she is isolated from them. The illustrations used are a pen-and-ink sketch of her state upon admission, and a drawing from a photograph of the recovered A. T. three months later. The images serve the self-congratulatory function of illustrating the success of Dowse's regime: 'The cure was unquestionably brought about by the administration of fluid nourishment'. Although Dowse refrains from forced feeding, the girl is given little choice but to eat as tube feeding is used 'frequently' as a threat; her food refusal is defeated with the use of egg and milk cocktails and plenty of beef tea.[32]

No. 1.

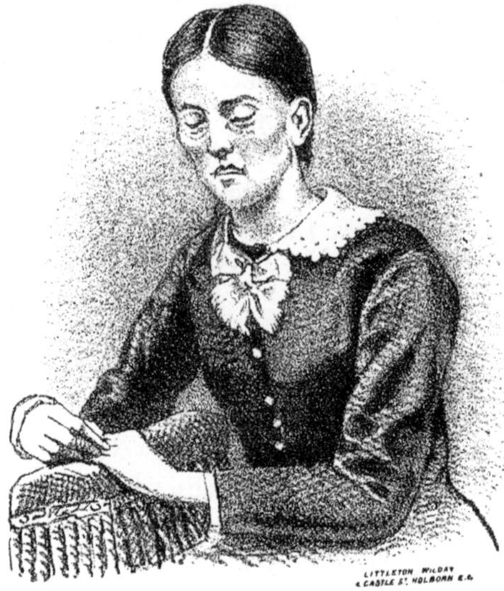

Drawn from pen and ink sketch, showing state of patient before treatment.

No. 2.

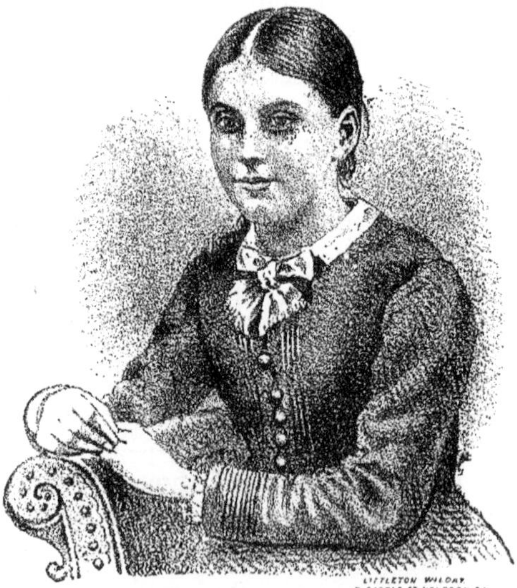

Drawn from the original photograph, showing the state of the patient after treatment

Figure 5.4: A. T., in T. Stretch Dowse, 'Anorexia Nervosa', *Medical Press and Circular*, 17 August 1881, pp. 95–7, 147–8, on p. 147. Wellcome Library, London.

Dowse is enthusiastic about this regime: 'her condition upon her admission and upon her departure was very *striking* and characteristic'. The images fit the narrative gloss of the case so well that it is as if they were commissioned to illustrate this point. The patient upon admission is 'unable to stand without assistance' with 'eyes downcast' and looks 'the picture of misery'. She is 'taciturn, shy and reserved', arrested in 'a general morbid state of functional inactivity'. Of particular note are the eyes: they are closed, and marked with heavy shadows, making her head appear skull-like. The head is inclined, and she appears to lean on the chair for support, her thin fingers and bony wrists protruding from her dress. The gaunt, hollow cheeks and morose expression complete the look of 'misery', and these details all connote refusal of the male gaze which seeks pleasure in displays of normative femininity. This eschewing of social engagement is reflected in Dowse's observations, too, for he focuses on the strangeness of her look: 'the extremities were cold and of a bluish colour ... the pupils of the eyes were sluggish, and did not contract readily to light'.[33] The coldness, the unresponsive eyes and the movement away from her observer suggest a position of retreat, a subversive refusal to engage in social rituals such as eating.

Although not unkind, Dowse is clear that in his view sympathy and understanding are not what are required. He equates recovery with the doctor's control over the patient's will: 'It is really astonishing to see with what remarkable rapidity these apparently hopeless and helpless causes are restored to perfect health when they are placed under proper and appropriate treatment, *even when death seems inevitable*'. The emphasis on the power of death reveals the seriousness of the threat posed by anorexia, and Dowse admits his own weakness when faced with a food-refuser: 'I have found myself *powerless* to do my patient any good whilst she has been subject to the sympathy and irresolute action of her immediate friends'.[34] The image of recovery functions as a comforting antidote to the horror of impotence. A. T. is now depicted with rounded cheeks, eyes alert and engaged and holding herself up with her own strength. She is visibly smiling, and her head is raised. All this confirms Dowse's final assessment: 'Instead of being taciturn and reserved, she was cheerful and agreeable to all around her, and took her food without any reserve or hesitation'.[35] In none of these cases are we offered any follow-up information about the continued health of the patient, so we are left wondering if this striking transformation could possibly be maintained. The addiction to anorexia so often proves to have stronger staying power than any treatment, as illustrated by the DSM-IV statistics, and these images of 'recovery' appear as naïve illustrations of the doctors' powerful fantasy of integrity and control that is imperfectly but neatly imposed onto an uncontrollable body. They illustrate a level of scopophilic pleasure by simultaneously satisfying the medical narrative of cure and the male bourgeois gaze by returning to an image of feminine normality.

The next case, Miss K. R., is presented in Gull's 1888 and 1894 articles using the same 'before' image but different 'after' pictures (Figures 5.5 and 5.6). Gull is concerned to give visual evidence of an unusual case: 'The case was so extreme that, had it not been photographed and accurately engraved, some assurance would have been necessary that the appearances were not exaggerated, or even caricatured, which they were not'.[36] Gull's paper serves to demonstrate his unique ability to bring young women such as these from the brink of death back to normal functioning, without delving into the murky business of their states of mind. In this sense, his reporting is optimistic and reassuring of the power of the physician to heal, and the images used appear to support this view. However, the pictures also reveal much that is meaningful in the attitude of patients towards their treatment.

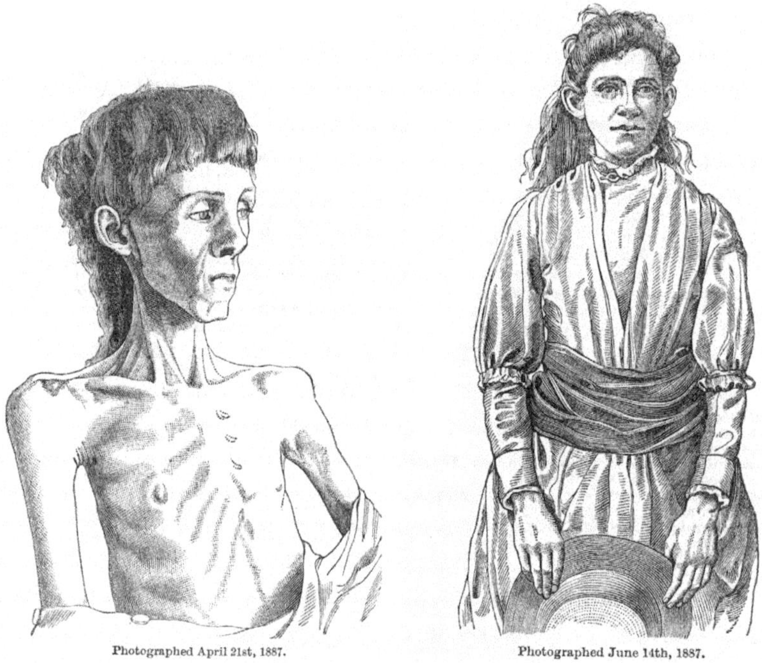

Figure 5.5: Miss K. R. ('before' and 'after' picture), in Gull, 'Anorexia Nervosa', *Lancet*, 131 (1888), pp. 516–17. Wellcome Library, London.

Miss K. R. is depicted in a posture of defiance, eyes averted and head turned away as if refusing to be captured or pinned down, her lips pursed in a gesture of closing off and her arms crossed defensively. She appears to embody the insubordination, the 'perversions of the "ego"', identified by Gull.[37] Her hair is cut into a brutally short, boyish fringe and is awkwardly pulled back. She is the only one of Gull's patients to be pictured naked; her breasts are flat, and she appears fragile, childlike and androgynous. The recovery image of Miss K. R. depicts her clothed in a billowing dress: this accentuates her fuller form and shows that she has undergone a process of feminization. Her hair is lifted from her face and flows loosely at the back, suggesting volume and health in contrast to the harsh and unwieldy style of the previous picture. Her arms hang down, holding a hat in a gesture of humility; the removal of her hat for the photograph also suggests that there is a social interaction going on between viewer and subject. These details combined suggest the patient accepts that she must behave like a middle-class girl of the period. Typical examples of paintings and portrait photographs of well-to-do young women from the period, such as Édouart Manet's 1872 portrait, *Berthe Morisot with a Bouquet of Violets*, and the photographer Carjat's 1886 portrait of the sculptor Camille Claudel reveal such details as hats, neatly styled hair, brooches, gloves, full skirts and carefully controlled posture to be important signs of respectable womanhood. Through these details of dress and hairstyle, modesty and passivity are equated with feminine normality as well as physical and mental health. The narrative emphasis on recovery suppresses completely the passive-aggressive psychological position represented by food refusal, and overlays these subversive 'before' images with new ones that conform to the expectations of the male gaze. In Gull's 1894 paper, the same 'before' image is used but a different 'after' image has been chosen (Figure 5.6). In the later paper, the recovered Miss K. R. is shown in a half-body shot, still naked – although notably fleshier – with the same flowing hair and half-smile. This later image accentuates the medical success of the feeding regime, whereas the clothed image supports the moral message of the correction of rebellious behaviour and the re-adoption of normal middle-class, Victorian feminine habits.

These recovery images typically reveal attitudes that are pleasing to doctors: dignity and compliance with Victorian social codes, illustrated by the engagement with the viewer's gaze. Brumberg, who briefly analyses Gull's images, observes:

> In all of the 'before' pictures there was a look of derangement, a look that was not present in the 'after' portraiture, where the girls looked tranquil, pleasant and ordinary. In their healthy state, each of the girls ... assumed the demeanour proper to young women of their role and station and lost the look of dour petulance that Gull believed characterized the anorectic.[38]

The picture of health demonstrates not only an end to the rebellion, but a rationale for carrying out treatment that could be brutal and that was often implemented against the will of the patient. On the one hand, they show doctors' need to be gratified and, on the other, the anorectic's desire to please.

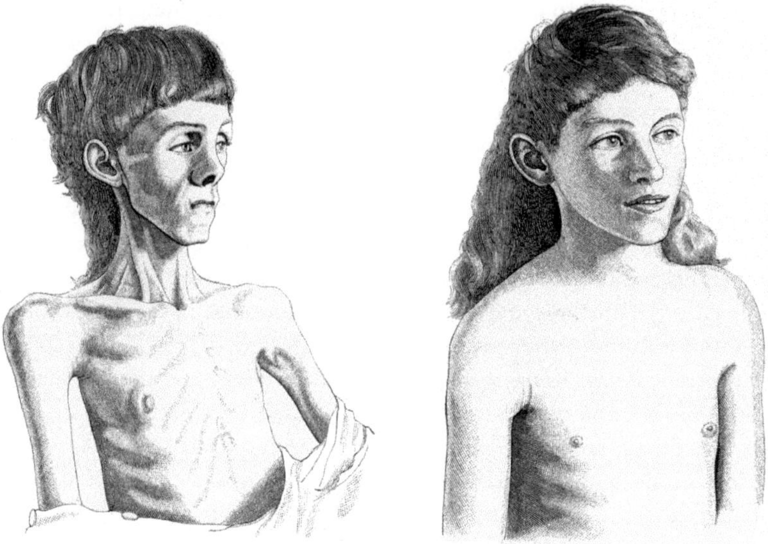

Photographed April 21st, 1887. Photographed June 14th, 1887.[1]

Figure 5.6: Miss K. R. ('before' and alternative 'after' picture), in Gull, 'Anorexia Nervosa' (1894), pp. 312–13. Wellcome Library, London.

The brutality of forced feeding is matched only by the harshness with which the anorectic treats her own body. As Bruch would later observe: 'In many ways these girls treat themselves as if they were slave labourers, who are denied all pleasures and indulgences and are fed a minimum of food and driven to work to the point of physical exhaustion'.[39] This extreme over-compliance with the expectation that she, as a woman, be self-effacing and passive, the subtlety and complexity of her position, is missed by commentators like Gull whose simplistic gloss of the case appears brutish and heavy-handed by comparison. The paradoxical elusiveness of her position is revealed, however, in her image.

Following in Lasègue's footsteps, in 1894 Drs Brissaud and Souques presented a similar case of recovery from anorexia in the Parisian medical journal the *Nouvelle Iconographie de la Salpêtrière*.[40] Their patient is photographed from behind in a rather intimate pose, her bottom half shrouded by a sheet and top half naked (Figure 5.7). This position illustrates a harrowing contrast between the visible bones – shoulder blades, ribs, vertebrae – of the first image and the fleshiness of the 'after' shot. In the first, the patient's hands are gripping a chair, which draws attention to her long, stick-like digits and, as with Dowse's weak patient, suggests fragility and dependency. The authors' stated purpose is 'to demonstrate how far the *delusion of thinness* can go'.[41]

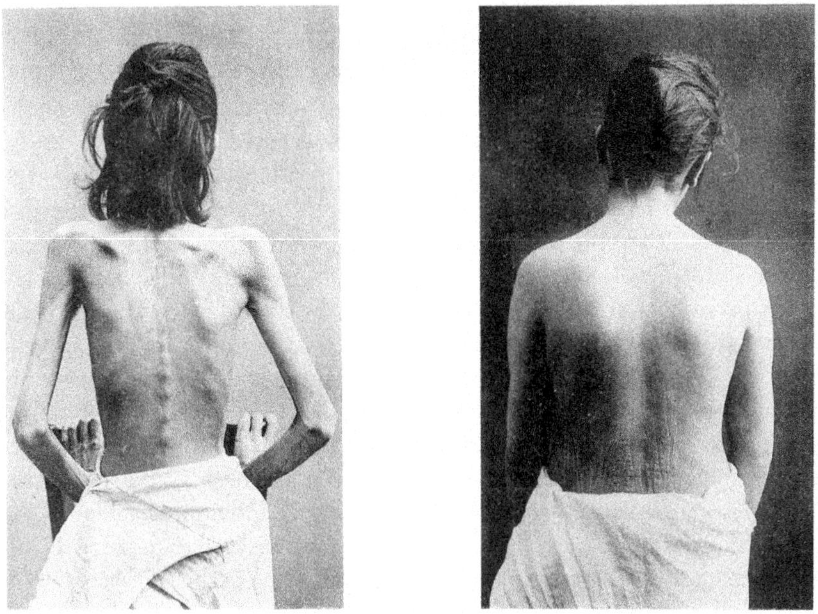

Avant le traitement. Après le traitement.

DÉLIRE DE MAIGREUR CHEZ UNE HYSTÉRIQUE

Figure 5.7: Julie R., in E. Brissaud and A. Souques, 'Délire de maigreur chez une hystérique', *Nouvelle Iconographie de la Salpêtrière*, 7 (1894), pp. 327–37, on p. 334. Wellcome Library, London.

The case history presented involves the doctor's battle with a constellation of troubling behaviours: the nineteen-year-old patient, 'Julie R.', suffers from extreme bulimia as well as anorexia, her vomiting being repeatedly described, in combative terms, as 'incessant, irrepressible'.[42] Compared to the English case studies, the French doctors seem greatly concerned with examining the patient's altering psychological states. Brissaud and Souques include a lengthy discussion of the issue of guilt and punishment, for Julie R. believed her illness was divine punishment for not having confessed the sin of masturbation. She experiences liminal states – between dreaming and hallucination – where she sees herself thrown into hell. Whilst there is some attempt made to understand the psychology of the patient, these semi-delusional religious beliefs and crippling guilt are construed as things that need to be corrected rather than explored. In order to achieve this, the doctors reflect back to the patient 'the futility of her ideas', and use forced feeding as a threat if she does not eat 'willingly'.[43] The patient's physical recovery is paralleled with the achievement of control over her will: 'The delusions of guilt and damnation no longer exist. The patient can remember them clearly, and now understands how futile they are.'[44] There is a semantic slippage in French between the 'inanition' of the body and the 'inanité' (futility, pointlessness) of the patient's beliefs, which are as thin and insubstantial as the body. In this sense, the layering of flesh on the body illustrated in the photographs reflects the numbing of the mind that being cured entails.

The problem with the 'recovery' approach is that it confuses enforced weight gain with true recovery, and fails fully to appreciate the problem of relapse. Whilst the health of the patient is the clinical priority, these case studies neatly impose a superficial – but pleasurable – image of recovery onto a complex and unruly psychological state. Images serve a specific clinical agenda, and doctors' interpretations reveal more about that schema than about the roots of anorexic behaviour. However, images of illness reveal attitudes that kick against the expectations of doctors and parents and demonstrate the force of a compulsive behaviour that lies beyond absolute medical control. These case studies powerfully illustrate Gilman's idea that images of disease and health serve the purpose of suppressing anxiety about human vulnerability to and limited ability to cure illness; the gendered nature of the images also reveals a concern to correct a subversive image by overlaying it with one that is satisfying to the male gaze.

Narratives of Anxiety

The second group of case studies report either fatal or otherwise unsuccessful outcomes, and the photographing of the patient serves to distance the viewer from the diseased subject. In this sense, the anxiety aroused in the viewer is projected onto the image rather than the viewer using the image to suppress anxiety. Doctor's commentaries accompanying the images admit feelings of helplessness and horror when faced with this disease, and in the French cases the power of the image is intensified through the inexplicable practice of obscuring the patient's face, thereby to some extent suppressing the gaze of both viewer and object, because the eyes of the person being looked at cannot be seen. This curious practice also sets up a voyeuristic vantage point, for the viewer's perspective is hidden behind the mask in the same way that the anorectic's self-conscious look is suppressed: there is a loss of visual dialogue between viewer and patient. The removal of the patient's perspective makes these images voyeuristic, and yet the absence of images of recovery makes these cases even more troubling and potentially subversive of the male gaze, because at no point do they conform to its expectations.

The anonymizing of patients by blocking out the eyes is common practice today in clinical illustrations of disfiguring illnesses, but these cases seem to be unique in the nineteenth-century clinical literature. The *Nouvelle Iconographie* and the *Revue photographique des hôpitaux de Paris* reproduced many photographs of patients, often completely naked, suffering from a range of distressing illnesses.[45] Yet my research did not uncover a single example of a patient, other than an anorectic, whose face or eyes has been obscured in this way. We cannot know the exact reasons why this was done, but it produces two important effects: first, it singles out anorexia nervosa as something unique, whether singularly interesting or troubling; second, it dehumanizes the body and renders it 'uncanny' in the Freudian sense.

Freud says the feeling of the uncanny, a sense of 'familiar strangeness', is aroused by something that should remain repressed coming into awareness, perhaps in an unwelcome way.[46] In his analysis of Hoffmann's short story, 'The Sandman', Freud locates the source of this feeling in the anxiety caused by the threat of losing one's eyes. Predictably, perhaps, Freud interprets this as part of an Oedipal drama and his reading might be seen as reductive for this reason. It is, however, an extremely useful idea when considering these images that are 'made strange' by both the suppression of the eyes/gaze and by the way in which the body appears recognizable and yet also horrifying in its emaciation. Part of this horror is caused by the body's nascent sexuality being violently rejected by the food-refusing girl, but at the same time pushed forward by the body itself in its own refusal to be repressed. This is particularly evident in the disturbing juxtaposition, frequently observable and discussed in the following case studies, of an emaciated and child-like body with fully developed breasts.

Dr Wallet reported on two illustrated cases in the *Nouvelle Iconographie* in 1892 (Figures 5.8 and 5.9).[47] His first case pictured is a half-body shot of a naked woman photographed from front and back. In the photograph where she faces the camera, her face is obscured awkwardly by a hashing pattern suggestive of a mask or prison-like mesh. In the second case, the girl's face is not fully obscured but her eyes are awkwardly scratched out. Wallet describes the visual impact of his first patient as 'a surprising [*étonnante*] aesthetic aberration', recalling the common French translation of Freud's '*Unheimlich*' (uncanny) as '*inquiétante étrangeté*' – literally, a 'worrying strangeness'.[48] The cases of Miss B. and Miss V. present inconclusive outcomes: both gain a little weight under treatment but do not fully recover. Miss B. is shown in a half-body shot, naked, with her face obscured but her rounded breasts visible as a sign of sexual development. Her nakedness, paired with the removal of a recognizable face, like the hooded figure of one condemned to death connotes loss of dignity, alienation and shame. In common with many anorectics, Miss B. has an irrepressible urge to physical movement. Her frenetic walks around the grounds of the hospital are banned, and she is confined to her room. Even then she continues with a frenzied exercise regime, to which the doctor responds by committing her to bed and by 'removing her clothes'.[49] The stripping of the patient here resembles the act of photographing her: both are attempts to fix and restrain her.

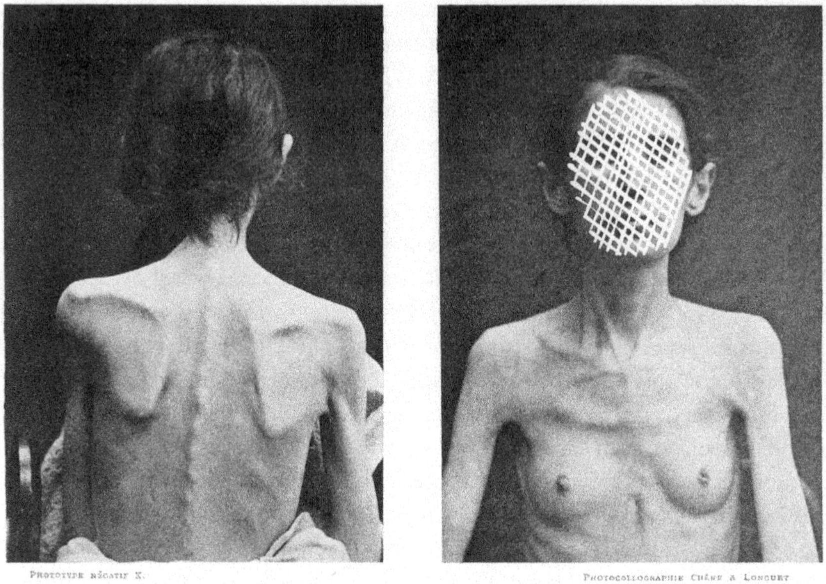

Figure 5.8: Miss B., in H. Wallet, 'Deux cas d'anorexie hystérique', *Nouvelle Iconographie de la Salpêtrière*, 5 (1892), pp. 276–80, on p. 276. Wellcome Library, London.

The theme of control is also invoked in the commentary on Miss V. She describes the anorexic behaviour as if it is an external power acting on her body which she is powerless to resist: 'It's as though there's a force that stops me when I want to eat'. This emerges as a destructive force of self-annihilation, urging Miss V. to drink vinegar and anything 'bad for the stomach'.[50] In a reversal of the pattern shown in the first group of studies, the healthy image shown is the one prior to anorexia and treatment rather than an image of recovery, exposing the violence inflicted on the body by self-starvation. The anorexic Miss V. appears sullen, tentatively lowering her nightdress to reveal emaciated shoulders. The subtle details of the image of sickness – a slightly hunched posture; hollow, expressionless eyes; a brooding expression – betray both vulnerability and resistance to social pressures. Miss V. is performing her illness, confirming stereotypes of feminine fragility, but paradoxically refusing to be bound by expectations of normality. Constantly cold, she wraps herself delicately in mittens and woollen tights even in the summer months – these layers of wrapping functioning as a symbolic flesh to cover her bony frame and to mitigate her vulnerability.

A fatal case of anorexia was reported by Lockhart Stephens, chief medical officer of the Emsworth Cottage Hospital near Bristol, in the *Lancet* in 1895 (Figure 5.10). It reproduces two striking woodcut illustrations based on photographs of the patient at the point of death.[51] Stephens describes a rather sullen

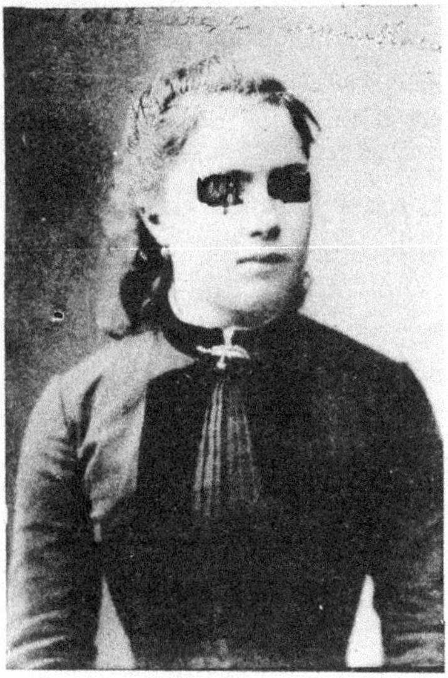

Fig. 1

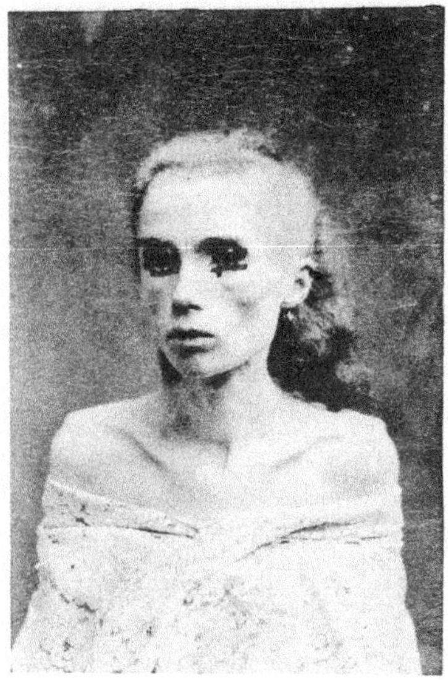

Fig. 2

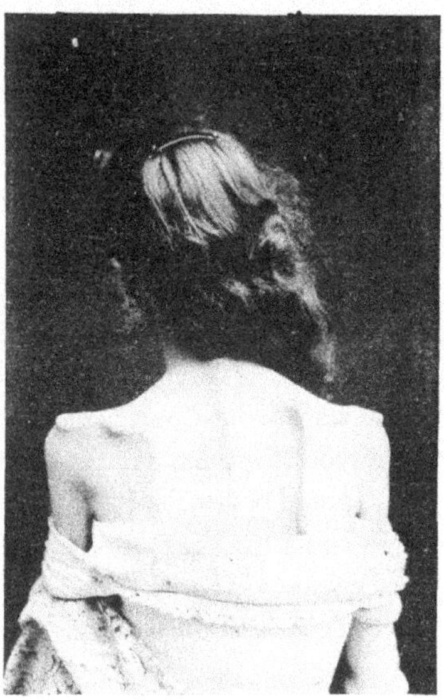

Fig. 3

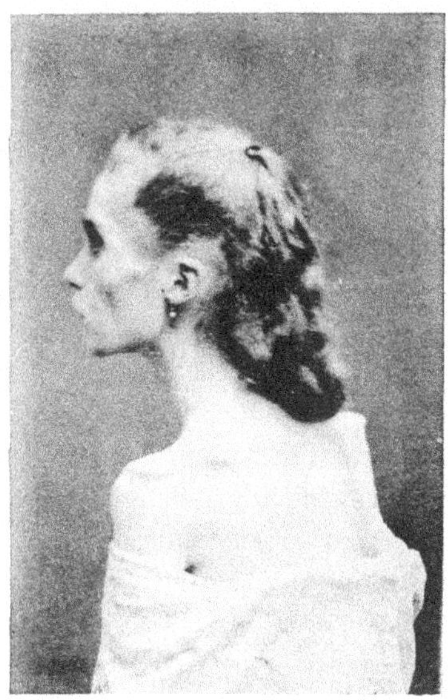

Fig. 4

Figure 5.9: Miss V., in Wallet, 'Deux cas d'anorexie hystérique', p. 278. Wellcome Library, London.

and manipulative girl, 'the spoilt child of the family', whose mother was 'quite under the influence of the patient'. Presenting the patient as an attention seeker, the clinical narrative moves swiftly from a picture of an initially compliant – although fretful – patient to a detailed clinical description of her rapid decline and death. Despite orders to keep her in bed 'with limbs and body bandaged in cotton wool' and 'to be fed every four hours', it seems that intervention simply came too late.[52] The girl is depicted lying on her deathbed, and in mortality there is a significant difference in the effect of the image on the viewer. The girl's eyes are visibly roving in different directions, representing the loss of engagement with the viewer's gaze, in contrast to the powerful, deliberately averted gaze of anorectics who hang on to life. The loss of self-consciousness in death reveals an acutely voyeuristic fascination with the anorexic body, for there can be no hope of reversing her symptoms, and the predominant interest lies in her sickness and death rather than in the pleasure of the recovered body. The girl simply looks like a victim of the ravages of starvation, consumed entirely and utterly defeated. Gone is the defiance and glowering moodiness evoked earlier in the story: there is no attitude left because she has finally effaced herself. This reinforces the previous observation made about the potency of the anorexic gaze. This patient's head lolls limply to the side, and despite her lightness her arms lie heavily on the bed. The second image evokes Christ-like suffering, as though she is lying in a tomb wrapped in grave clothes. As with the other cases, the stubborn breasts are the only remaining signs of life: 'The body was extremely emaciated; there was not a trace of fat in the subcutaneous tissue with the exception of the breasts, which stood out boldly'.[53]

The significance of the dead body being photographed in this way may be compared to the more general voyeuristic fascination with the female corpse in contemporary works of art. A particularly relevant intertext to consider is the Austrian Gabriel von Max's painting *Der Anatom* (1869) which depicts an anatomist poised over the body of a beautiful young woman in a moment of hesitation before carrying out the dissection of her body.[54] Like Lockhart Stephens's patient, the body is shrouded and laid out for the purposes of medical observation. As with many of the anorexic images discussed here, a prominent detail of the painting is an apparently unnaturally raised and subtly exposed breast. This, combined with the gaze of her medical observer being contained within the painting, lends the painting an erotic charge that is not straightforwardly present in the anorexic images discussed here. However, Elisabeth Bronfen argues that the woman's body is presented as being perfected in death:

> The moment von Max has chosen to arrest in his painting is one where beauty is defined in contrast to destruction ... The painting enacts a crucial moment of hesitation: the draping of the shroud underscores the aesthetisation by suggesting the

> materialisation of a statue. The feminine body appears as a perfect, immaculate aesthetic form because it is a dead body, solidified into an object of art.[55]

When considering Bronfen's observations, what strikes us about the anorexic images is that, compared to the conventional aestheticization of the dead female body, the destruction of the perfect female form takes place during the life of the subject: even if it causes the end of her life, the process of dying coincides with the last stages of life in which the anorexic woman is corpse-like. In this sense, the destruction of the 'perfect, immaculate' feminine body appears as a profoundly subversive act because it is carried out by the woman herself. It makes the almost-dead female body *un*feminine, ugly, horrifying and yet still fascinating.

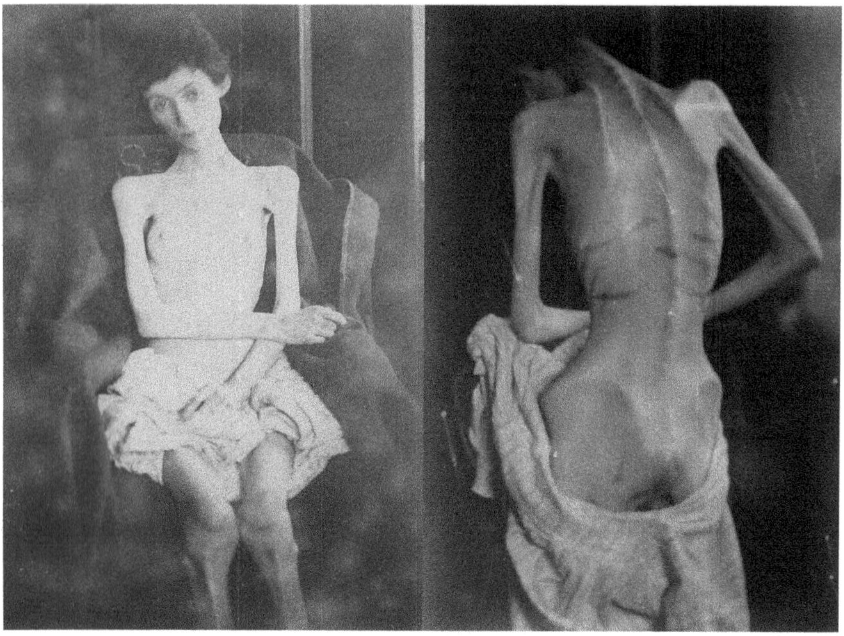

Figure 5.11: St Bartholomew's Hospital Archives and Museum patient. Front view and back view, 1896, St Bartholomew's Hospital Archives and Museum, London, SBHU MU/14/49/16/1, 2, Wellcome Images. Wellcome Library, London.

There is also an 1896 image of an anorexic patient held in St Bartholomew's Hospital Archives and Museum, without accompanying case notes (Figure 5.11).[56] In the rear view, the patient is struggling to stand and resembles an exoskeletal insect, with bones painfully protruding beneath a stretched layer of waxy, diaphanous skin. The buttocks have taken on the familiar concave shape; the lowered nightdress resembles a grave shroud and the bent posture suggests shame and physical frailty, as though she is an elderly woman. Pictured from the front, the seventeen-year-old patient sits with her head slightly lowered and inclined, with her arm crossed over her lap as if to reduce the level of exposure. Her seated

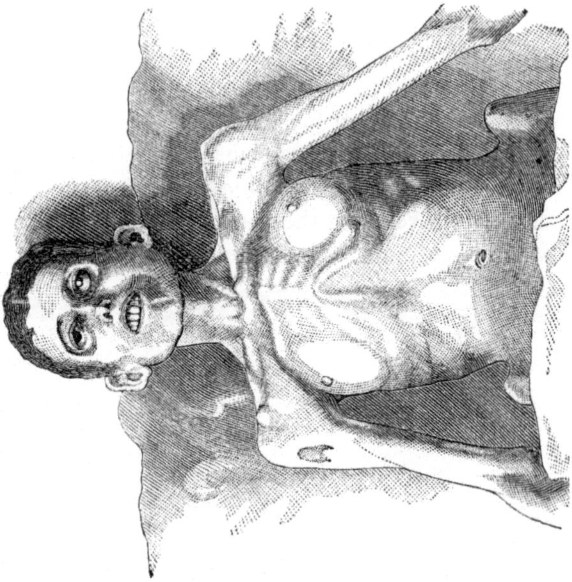

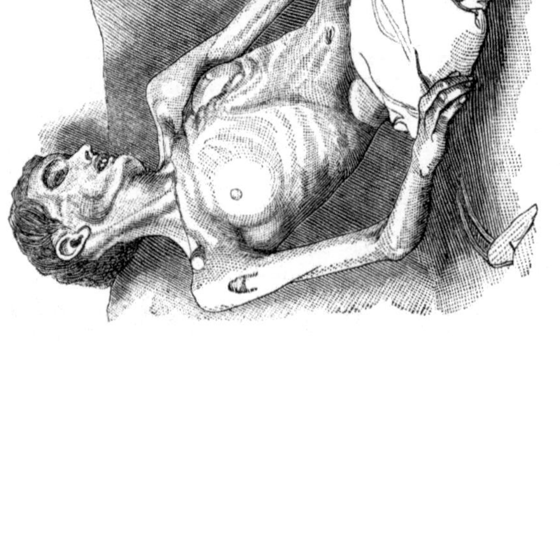

position seems to be a defensive one in which she is trying to conceal herself and her evident discomfort at being photographed. The enigmatic look she projects carries a wealth of potential interpretations: uncomfortable, and yet also defiant and stubborn. She locks the viewer's gaze with hypnotic strength by staring directly at her observer, suggesting a powerful defiance of medical scrutiny and a potently passive-aggressive attitude to her developing body – confirmed by the fullness of the breasts observed previously.

The case of sixteen-year-old Béatrice Gill was reported by Dr Georges Gasne, a clinical consultant in nervous illnesses at the Salpêtrière, in the *Nouvelle Iconographie* in 1900 (Figure 5.12). Like his colleagues, Gasne blocks out the patient's face, insisting: 'we *have had to* obscure the face here'.[57] The fact that he makes this point suggests there would be a level of shame in being identified as an anorectic. Béatrice's appearance is described as 'horrifying'; she weighs just 55lb and Gasne remarks: 'one cannot imagine a more emaciated skeleton'.[58] Gasne's response, emphasizing the feeling of obligation in concealing this woman's identity alongside the 'horror' of her look, betrays a feeling of anxiety experienced by those pioneering treatment of this mysterious disease.

In the case report, the problematic nature of feeding and food is invoked from birth. We are told that Béatrice was initially bottle fed, but at four months became 'malnourished', needing to be 'put to the breast' – presumably that of a wet nurse. Separated from her mother, she began to grow.[59] But once returned Béatrice 'failed to thrive until the age of four' and it would seem that her family stifled her growth, right from birth.[60] The question as to why her mother could not or would not nurse her child – artificial feeding being almost certainly fatal even in the late nineteenth century – is not asked, but Béatrice's early years are marked by the fragmentation of her emotional attachments and by multiple disruptions in the caregiving environment.[61] Such interesting background details are conspicuously absent from English case reports.

Gasne's commentary is inflected with intense ambivalence, a tension between the horror of the image and the reality of the patient. On the one hand, his genuine captivation with the patient is revealed in the adjectives 'gay', 'emotional', 'gentle' and 'sensitive'; yet on the other hand, Béatrice's appearance evokes dread.[62] When dressed, we are told, Béatrice strikes her observer with her 'slenderness' and 'youthfulness'. But her naked, photographed form presents the unsettling paradox of hideous, skeletal features alongside full breasts, unaffected by the emaciation, which Gasne calls 'remarkable': 'If it had not been for the conservation of the mammary glands in this young girl (*remarkable* under the circumstances), it could really be said that she was reduced to just skin and bones'. So Gasne emphasizes her sexual development, but her skeletal form also troubles him – her face in particular. In contrast to the previous depiction, her face is said to be 'utterly haggard', giving her 'the look of an old woman'.[63] These paradoxical allusions recall Gull's suggestion that the anorexic body is somehow out of harmony with its real age: child-like, adolescent and yet also like a post-menopausal woman.

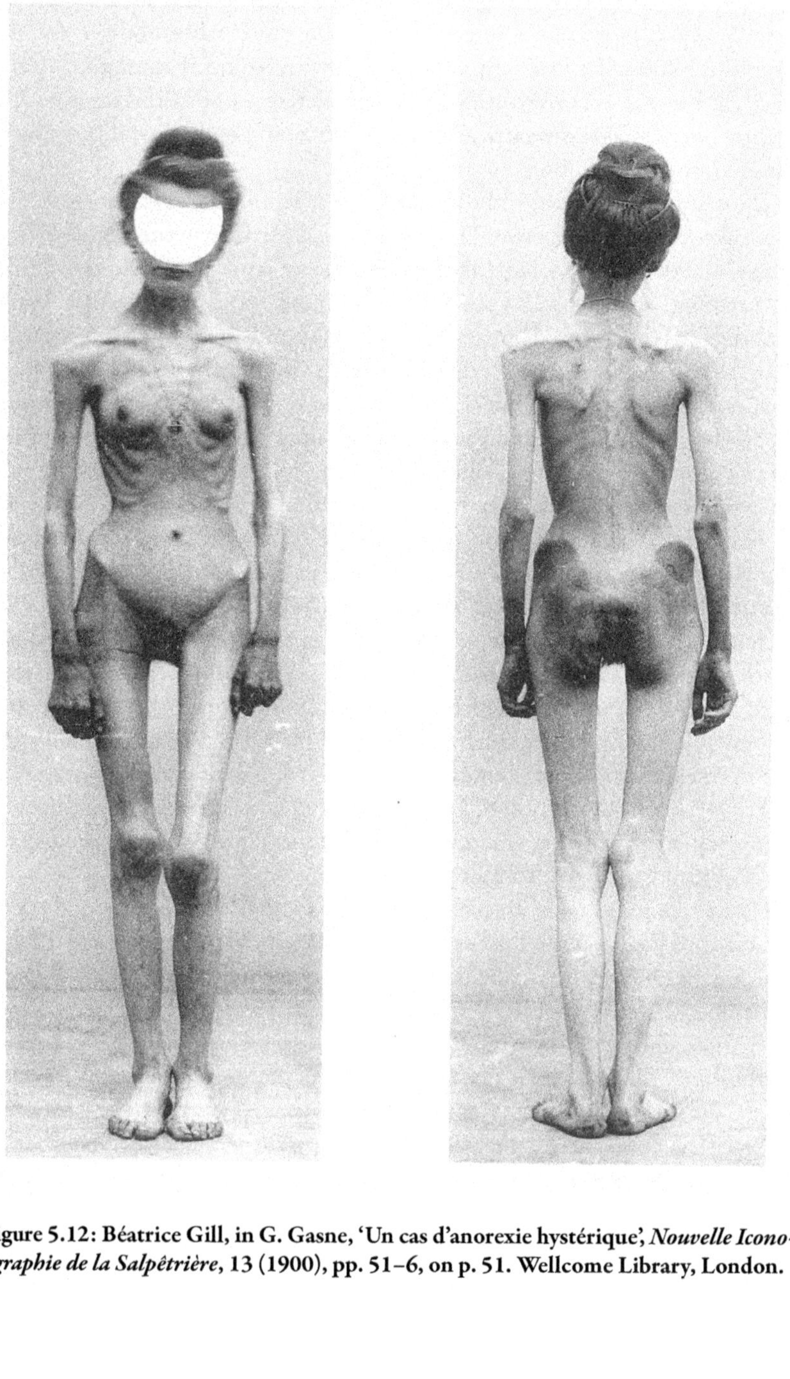

Figure 5.12: Béatrice Gill, in G. Gasne, 'Un cas d'anorexie hystérique', *Nouvelle Iconographie de la Salpêtrière*, 13 (1900), pp. 51–6, on p. 51. Wellcome Library, London.

This is a body in conflict with itself. Gasne says these troublesome breasts seem not to fit the emaciated body, 'the voluminous breasts stand out'. The breasts present an enigma for both doctor and patient, and are an illustration of the paradox of the body being hyper-controlled and yet recalcitrant: the body is determined to grow, but Béatrice is resolute in her attempt to stunt it. Despite never having menstruated, Béatrice's uncomfortable breasts act as a physical reminder of the latent forces of puberty: 'her breasts are *always* a little painful and the patient is *always* afraid of them being knocked'.[64] The repetition of this adverb reinforces the idea of the troublesome nature of her body. Gasne concludes his case study by noting regretfully that his patient relapsed soon after leaving hospital, and does not seem overly concerned with the question of her 'cure'. This suggests a level of voyeurism in his preoccupation with the strangeness of her sick body, which interests him most when he can gaze upon it.

A decade after Gasne's discussion of the disease, a young Dr Nogues wrote a detailed medical thesis on anorexia, published in Toulouse in 1913. Somewhat unusually for a thesis, it contains two photographs of anorectics that represent the latest images in the French literature in the period under discussion.[65] Nogues is initially optimistic about the possibilities offered by modern treatment, citing Professor Déjerine in his introduction: 'The treatment of anorexia [*anorexie mentale*] is a type that gives excellent results'.[66] Despite this outlook, Nogues's two illustrated cases did not have positive results: Miss G. was another fatal case, and Miss M. C. became a chronic case.[67] Nogues fully admits the failure of medical treatment in both cases. Miss M. C. (Figure 5.13), who weighed just 18.7 kg (41lb) at her first admission, is the most extreme example of emaciation discussed in this essay. In the case of Miss M. C., Nogues says he feels impotent in attempting to untangle the enmeshed family relationships, calling himself 'completely helpless in the face of the patient's obstinacy' and the parents' weakness.[68] As with Lockhart Stephens, the doctors' sense of impotence is projected onto the parents who are routinely blamed for the failure of treatment.

Miss G. (Figure 5.14) is a patient who, as well as being anorexic, 'inflicts bodily punishments on herself'.[69] In line with the more sensitive appraisal of the patient's state of mind that accompanies the French case studies, the themes of guilt, punishment and sacrifice are underlined. Nogues reports that 'she believes that the devil inside her feeds on everything that she eats'.[70] This curious delusion functions as a powerful metaphor for the body consuming itself, and can be paralleled with the sense of mind–body dissociation evoked in the cases of Béatrice Gill and Miss V., who both describe the body as an autonomous agent bent on self-destruction. Miss G., profoundly affected by having witnessed her mother die in childbirth when she was just twelve, cannot ingest milk. Just as Béatrice failed to thrive on the milk offered by her mother, Nogues tells us that Miss G. dramatically vomits the very substance that symbolizes maternal sustenance, suggesting an involuntary rejection of the mother who abandoned her.

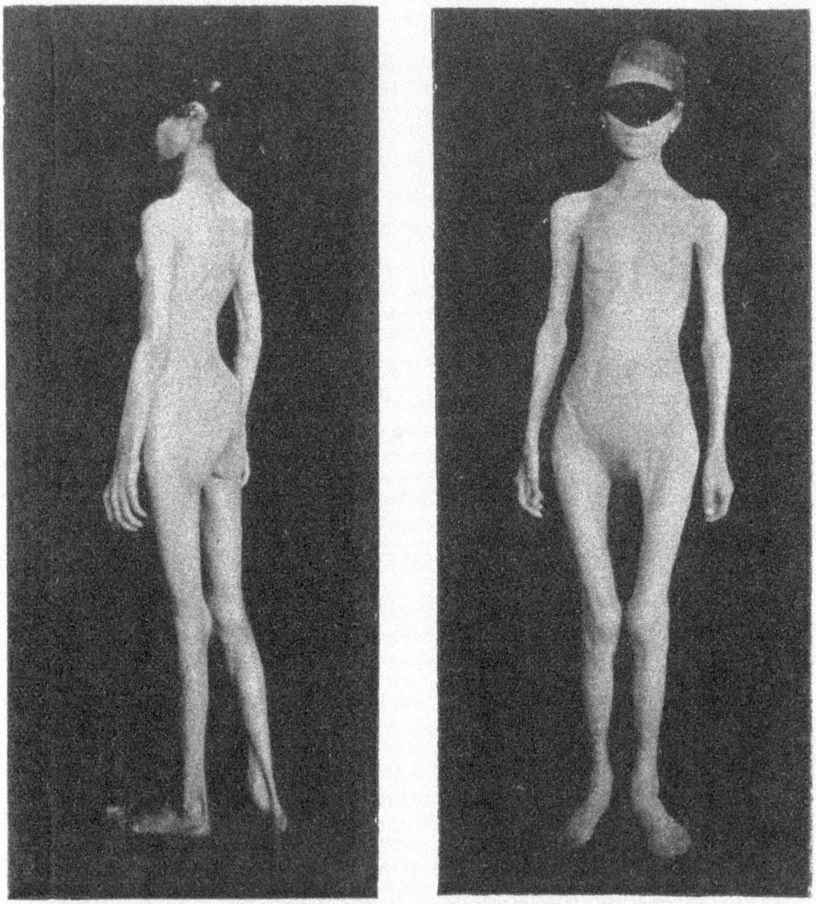

Figure 5.13: Miss M. C., in G. Noguès, *L'anorexie mentale et ses rapports avec la psycho-physiologie de la faim* (Toulouse: Dirion, 1913), pp. 149–58, on p. 154. Bibliothèque nationale de France.

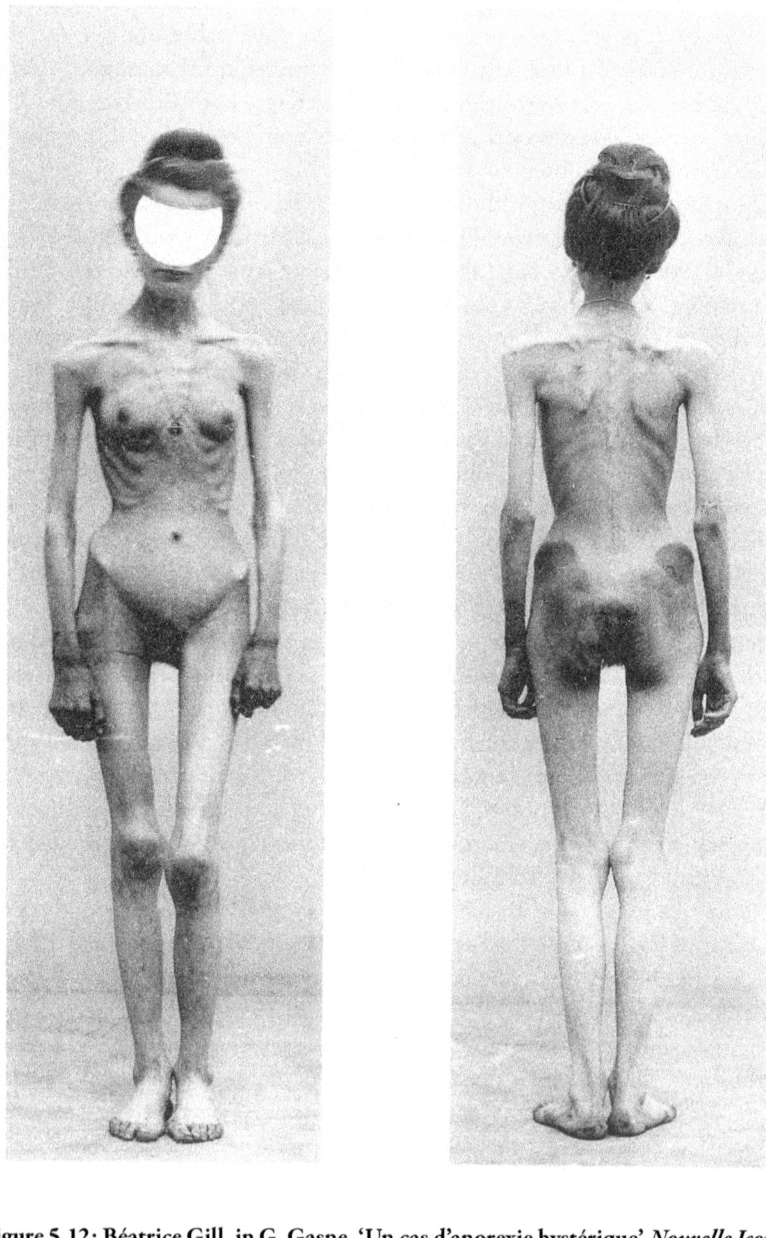

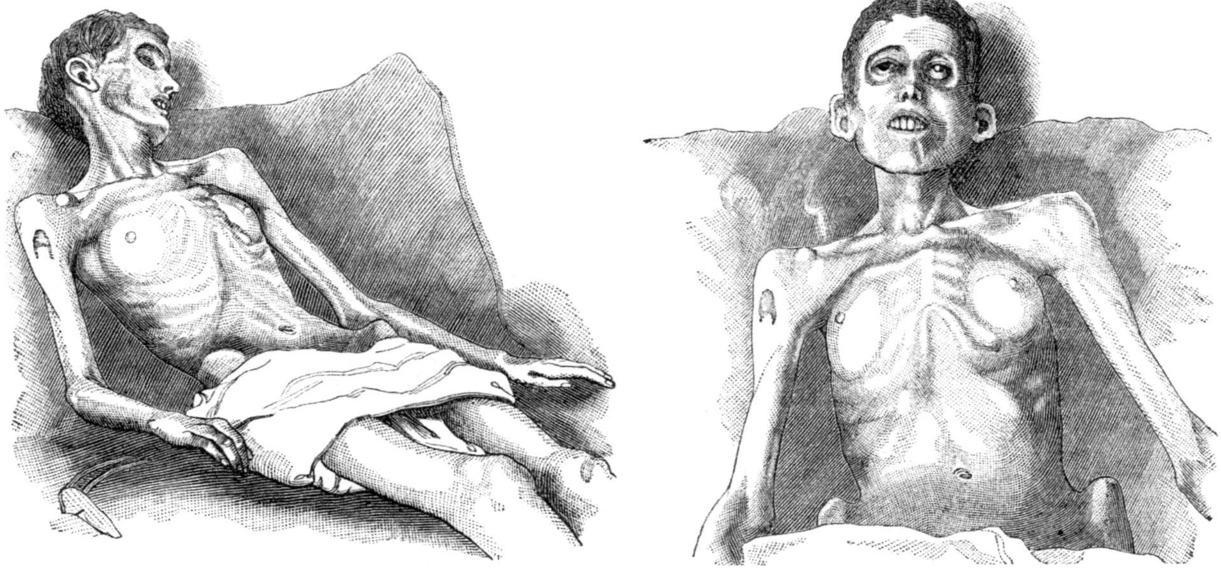

Figure 5.10: Lockhart Stephens's patient, in L. Stephens, 'Case of Anorexia Nervosa', *Lancet*, 145 (1895), pp. 31–2. Wellcome Library, London.

> materialisation of a statue. The feminine body appears as a perfect, immaculate aesthetic form because it is a dead body, solidified into an object of art.[55]

When considering Bronfen's observations, what strikes us about the anorexic images is that, compared to the conventional aestheticization of the dead female body, the destruction of the perfect female form takes place during the life of the subject: even if it causes the end of her life, the process of dying coincides with the last stages of life in which the anorexic woman is corpse-like. In this sense, the destruction of the 'perfect, immaculate' feminine body appears as a profoundly subversive act because it is carried out by the woman herself. It makes the almost-dead female body *un*feminine, ugly, horrifying and yet still fascinating.

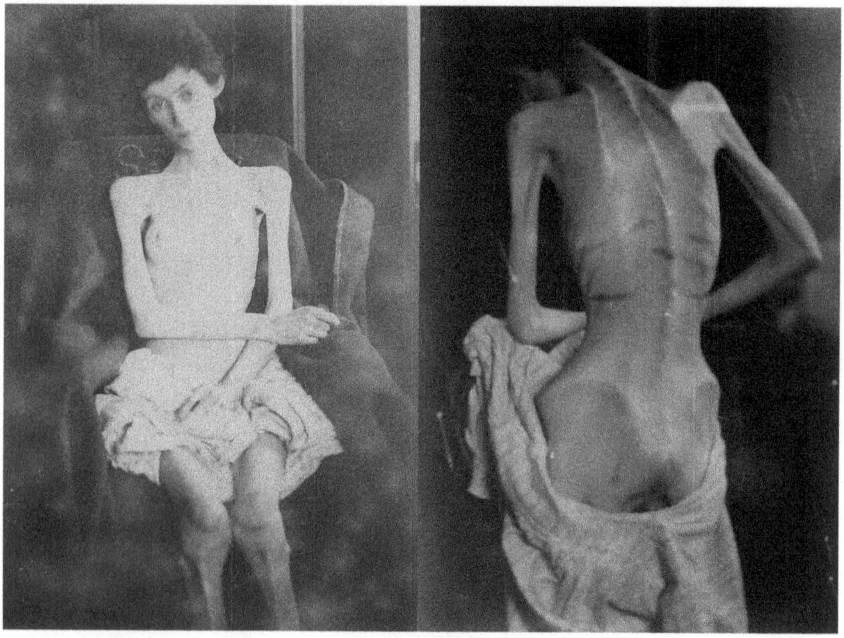

Figure 5.11: St Bartholomew's Hospital Archives and Museum patient. Front view and back view, 1896, St Bartholomew's Hospital Archives and Museum, London, SBHU MU/14/49/16/1, 2, Wellcome Images. Wellcome Library, London.

There is also an 1896 image of an anorexic patient held in St Bartholomew's Hospital Archives and Museum, without accompanying case notes (Figure 5.11).[56] In the rear view, the patient is struggling to stand and resembles an exoskeletal insect, with bones painfully protruding beneath a stretched layer of waxy, diaphanous skin. The buttocks have taken on the familiar concave shape; the lowered nightdress resembles a grave shroud and the bent posture suggests shame and physical frailty, as though she is an elderly woman. Pictured from the front, the seventeen-year-old patient sits with her head slightly lowered and inclined, with her arm crossed over her lap as if to reduce the level of exposure. Her seated

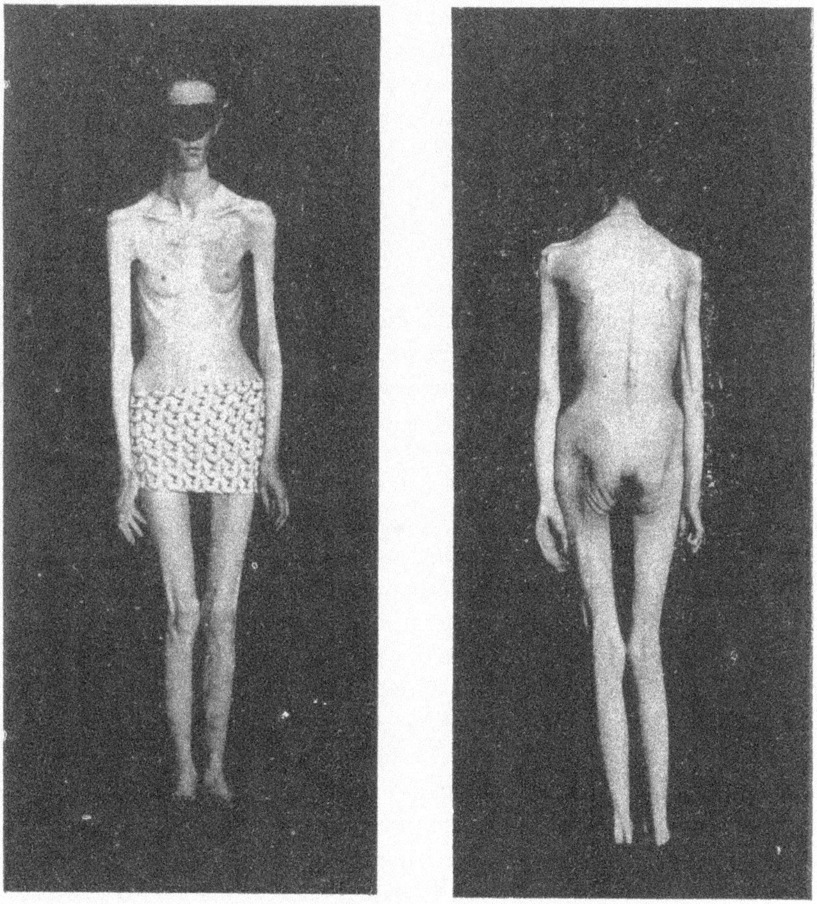

Figure 5.14: Miss G., in Noguès, *L'anorexie mentale et ses rapports avec la psychophysiologie de la faim*, pp. 159–62, on p. 160. Bibliothèque nationale de France.

The indistinct photograph of the patient shows that – despite her extreme emaciation – she is still able to stand, although her arms hang limply by her sides and her fingers seem to be clawing in discomfort. Her eyes obscured, the front view shows a shroud-like covering, which with her salient ribs announces her death. The presence of rounded breasts, like with Béatrice, stubbornly contrasts with painfully bony, concave buttocks enclosed in thin, sagging folds of skin. The case concludes with a detailed description of her decline and death, a story that is made more harrowing by the presence of such powerful images of resistance to treatment; the strength of these photographs contrasts markedly with the feeling of impotence expressed by those treating her. Like Dowse, who as we have already seen describes himself as 'powerless' when faced with a particularly intransigent patient, Noguès laments his patient's 'indomitable obstinacy'.[71]

In the final assessment, illustrations of patients appear to be important but little-studied records in the history of anorexia nervosa. The voyeuristic fascination with the disease, as identified in these early clinical documents, announces the twenty-first-century media obsession with excessively thin women. In the absence of a serious clinical attempt to understand the compulsive nature of anorexia, and in a context in which the voice of the patient is rarely heard, these images speak for the anorectic and to the viewer. The responses of the original viewers of these images are shot through with anxiety and conflicting feelings, due to the fact that they subvert the expectations of the heterosexual male gaze. Displaying these images served the dual purpose of containing and controlling a subversive behaviour that threatened the social order whilst at the same time distancing the threat posed by pathological conditions from the 'healthy' observer. In contrasting ways, male middle-class doctors and young, anorexic women conformed to the stifling and limiting values of their class. Their anxieties meet and are expressed in these case studies, in which men spoke textually and women spoke visually. Doctors attempted to speak for their patients by infantilizing them and insisting that they be placed under strong moral control. Unwittingly, however, they allowed these women to speak for themselves. The language of the patient's gaze is enigmatic and fleeting, but it is a communication that announces the more sensitive assessment of the meaning of anorexia that came later in the twentieth century with the psychoanalytical approaches pioneered by Hilde Bruch and Susie Orbach, who have made a concerted effort to understand that language. However, these images were at best only partially understood during their time; in a similar way, our culture's interest in images of very sick women is complex in its motivation. These nineteenth-century case studies may be read with a certain detachment afforded by hindsight, but we would do well, as a culture, to learn to question our own potentially voyeuristic treatment of this problem. As we have seen, the fascination with the sick body, as an end in itself, is demonstrated in the tendency we have to glamourize excessive thinness and objectify the female body.

6 KATE MARSDEN'S LEPER PROJECT: ON SLEDGE AND HORSEBACK WITH AN OUTCAST MISSIONARY NURSE

Tabitha Sparks

The 1892 travel memoir by missionary nurse Kate Marsden, *On Sledge and Horseback to the Outcast Siberian Lepers*, is at first glance a remarkable testimony to Marsden's 2,000 mile, ten-month journey across Russia and Siberia and back. The events Marsden narrates are so incredible, in fact, that since the time of the text's publication, readers have questioned its truthfulness. After the Siberian journey and the publication of the memoir, Marsden enjoyed a brief period of fame in England and beyond, winning the approval of luminaries including Queen Victoria, W. T. Stead and the Empress of Russia.[1] But rumours surrounding her work, particularly the management of the money she collected for her leper hospital and challenges to the veracity of the memoir soon eclipsed her celebrity status. Furthermore, the memoir's mixing of genres, changing objectives and focalizations all encode a textual version of the same unreliability that came to haunt Marsden's character and reputation. I will turn later, and briefly, to the contested afterlife of Marsden's memoir and the decline of her reputation, as what concerns this essay is the memoir itself. The prolific and contradictory objectives, voices and identities that constitute Marsden's memoir command attention beyond their likely exaggerations. Rather than consider Marsden alone in accounting for the memoir's textual incongruities, I relate them to the contradictory values and objectives of professional Victorian nursing as well.

Marsden's journey, she explains early in the text, was inspired by her experience as a nurse in the Russo-Turkish War of 1877, where she was first acquainted with the 'ravages' of leprosy. While in Constantinople and Tiflis she heard 'reports' of a Siberian herb that was said to 'alleviate the sufferings caused by leprosy, and in some cases, to remove the disease'.[2] These rumours convinced her to travel to Siberia and track down the herb, and eventually to nurse the neglected Siberian lepers themselves. In a broad sense the memoir follows this scheme, though the unnamed herb proves to be first elusive and later unverifiable.[3] By the memoir's end, the goal of nursing and treating the lepers has turned almost wholly into a campaign for funds on their behalf. When her journey is over, Marsden begins the process of building the lepers a hospital, which is erected in 1897 with money she has raised.[4] Thus, what begins as a medico-investigative journey ends as a fundraising endeavour. The memoir is followed by a lengthy appendix of documents attesting to Marsden's fundraising, outreach and benevolence, as well as to the hazards she faced on her journey.

In nineteenth-century studies and beyond, it has become conventional to read rhetorical complexity in women's texts (novels, autobiographies, travel journals, diaries) as discursive confirmations of women's liminal place in the literary marketplace and in public spheres more generally.[5] In many scholarly studies, textual ambiguity enables feminist scholars to find evidence of at least tacit resistance to the patriarchal system (whether literary, political, colonial) that can seem overdetermining.[6] The attribution of complexity or ambivalence to a text can challenge its clear allegiance to a belief system or discursive tradition and, by extension, can represent its authors' refusal to capitulate to convention. Much of this work is convincing and powerful, but as a methodological approach, it can also stop short of a commitment to an argument; an explanation of the text can be hedged by the proclamation of its hybridity. This essay attempts to go beyond the confirmation of Marsden's 'complexity' and 'contradictory discourses' to find some explanatory frame for them. Without question, Marsden's text is multivalent and inconsistent, but pointing that out and documenting it carefully does not have to be the end of the analysis.

Following the belief that all genres and formal features are socially entrenched, my proposed explanation of Marsden's discursive confusion is also social: I am exploring Marsden's vocation of nursing as a field that embodies the ambivalence so prominent in her memoir. Not nursing alone, moreover, but nursing as Marsden practices it – voluntary, missionary, dangerous. That the subjects she is nursing are lepers further qualifies her field: lepers at this time were incurable, contagious and usually grotesque. The first part of the essay focuses on the memoir's multiple discourses, drawing attention to two prevailing positions that Marsden occupies: the empowered, Christ-like saviour and the humble, unworthy servant. The memoir's numerous literary, rhetorical and political modes, as well as its formal features, more or less fit into these perspectival categories. The second part of the essay examines Marsden's representation of nursing in both ideological and formal contexts and also explores the literary and cultural history of the nurse that Marsden emulates. My aim, then, is to connect the text's discursive confusion to the mixed messages inherent in the role of the Victorian nurse that Marsden inherits and emulates.

Textual Complexity: From Empowerment to Debasement

A survey of the variegated literary and rhetorical modes in *On Sledge and Horseback* reveals how easily and often Marsden moves between oppositional subject positions; several of her discursive identities are heroic, powerful and authoritative, but others profess or exemplify meekness and subordination. The sheer number of dangers that Marsden faces and the number of times she fears for her life together invoke the late-century imperial romance. In H. Rider Haggard's *She* (1886–7), for instance, the intrepid (male) British travellers brave shipwreck, beheadings, a mutinous tribe; they traverse a bottomless crevasse over a flimsy plank; they escape the curse of immortality (but not the seduction of the African Queen, Ayesha). Like Haggard's heroes, Marsden represents herself as dedicated to a quest for which she willingly risks death. The dangers include feral wolves, bears and vividly described conditions ('The forest seemed on fire and the rain dashed in our faces with almost blinding force').[7] She narrowly survives accidents (in one she is 'snatched from the jaws of death' in a collision that maims her driver: 'his horrible, ghastly condition I dare not describe').[8] She fears the criminals whom she walks among in her prison visits ('I wondered they did not kill me in their desperation and how easily they could have done it!').[9] In addition to physical risk, Marsden faces the intrigues of political suspicion in a manner that evokes Kipling's spy-hero Kim who manoeuvres between the British secret service and native Indian operatives.[10] She prepares to 'battle' the 'jealously guarded' secret of the Siberian herb,[11] evoking the plot of a spy novel, a genre in which she also self-consciously participates: after a meeting with local dignitaries in Yakutsk, Marsden explains that '[n]ot withstanding my credentials, a suspicion existed that I was nothing better than a political spy'.[12] Hardy, self-reliant and determined, Marsden's evident comfort in a male sphere also aligns her with the late-century New Woman, as do her avowals of the difference between her journey and those undertaken by delicate 'lady tourists',[13] and the discomforts of the trip that made her feel 'more like a battered old log of mahogany than a gently nurtured Englishwoman'.[14] She starts the journey accompanied by a friend, Miss Field, who speaks Russian and acts as Marsden's companion. But illness forces Miss Field's return early on and so for much of the journey Marsden is 'the only woman' among a 'motley assemblage of men' (sledge drivers, guides, hosts, local officials).[15] She finds her singularity 'touching' but not improper, and makes many references to the masculine habits and clothing that conditions force her, cheerfully, to assume. These include 'adopting a man's mode of riding' and venturing to places where 'no English woman had ever visited'.[16] The contrast she draws between her own interests and those of her female friends further shows an eagerness to transcend the conventional portrait of femininity. She writes that she 'frequently irritated [her] friends when, in the midst of discussing things to wear and things to eat, [she] went off at a tangent to speak of the far-off lepers, and what they wanted'.[17] Like the New Women who worked to alter the political and professional horizon of Victorian women, Marsden has her eye on higher purposes than her 'lighthearted' friends.

As she reports them, Marsden's negotiations through Russia and Siberia force her into an imperially charged and authoritative position. This modality seems to obscure her gender behind the constructs of nation and race, as well as assumed economic status. Travelling towards Tobolsk, the residents of a small village implore Marsden to intervene with the government and stop the pollution of their river from a nearby paper mill. 'I certainly had not come to Siberia to look after polluted rivers', she writes, 'but how could I refuse to listen to their touching appeal?' Propelled by the 'reverence' of the villagers, Marsden showcases her diplomacy and visits the offending mill, meets with the Governor of Tobolsk, and alleges that he promises her to repair the problem.[18] After her return to Russia, Marsden begins her fundraising for the lepers in earnest, with ambitious goals. She targets 'all the leading people of Moscow and St. Petersburg on behalf of the lepers', and hopes to 'lay the sad state of their existence before Her Imperial Majesty the Empress'.[19] She subsequently extends these plans by saying that she 'hoped to establish a headquarters of a scientific society for investing the state of lepers and concerting measures for their relief wherever lepers existed throughout the Russian Empire'.[20]

Sara Mills has argued that most scholarship on Western women's travel writing underplay or neglect women's complicity with colonial politics;[21] it is more fashionable to align women with the repressed subject than with the colonial authority. While Russia and Siberia were not British colonies, they were also not 'the West', and their exoticism and primitivism to Marsden ('the natives [of Siberia], even now, are only in a semi-barbarous state, having but recently been brought under the influence of civilization')[22] as well as her background in colonial settings facilitate for my purposes their structural comparison to colonized nations. As well as Marsden's comfort with authority (or at least its representation), the imperial undertones of her project surface through her frequent assertions of English superiority. She disparages domestic conditions on her trip from the conscious perspective of English womanhood: '[b]eing an English woman, I was naturally pleased to see tempting butter once more, that had not been fingered and mauled by dirty peasants'.[23] Her critiques extend to government institutions and national character, too: the hospital in Tjumen was 'the worst [she had] ever seen', she writes, but explains that 'after my experience of clean, bright English hospitals, I am of necessity a severe critic'. She finds the kindly people in Krasnoyarsk much like 'British Colonials – frank, honest, upright, truthful and loyal. They will give a welcome to every stranger, and help all in need.'[24]

Beyond her novelistic heroism and imperialistic confidence, Marsden's evangelism consolidates her most vehement rhetorical stance, though she sometimes expresses her Christian subordination in language that is unconvincing. When, for instance, she offers the inmates of Tukalinsk prison tea and bread along with her usual distribution of religious tracts, she concedes that

> [s]ome friends might think that this trifling attention to the physical needs of the prisoners was superfluous, and that I ought to be contented with spiritual ministration. But I asked myself, I hope not presumptuously, what Christ would have done. And I felt that he would first attend in some degree to the material wants of such outcasts, before offering the Bread of Life ... I tried to reach their hearts by first attending to their bodies.[25]

The gesture to presumptuousness at least explicitly mitigates it, as we see in a similar account where Marsden bemoans the insistence of three Siberians who, within a four-page section of the text, all prostrate themselves before her, 'so unbounded was [their] gratitude'.[26] Elsewhere she abandons the pretense of humility and unselfconsciously invokes her influence: 'the reader can imagine, without my help, all that such outcasts are compelled to endure'; 'I know that today, in many a dwelling in Russia, both among rich and poor, prayers arise on my behalf to the Great Father of us all'.[27] Here she summarizes the objectives of her trip in one stunningly ambitious paragraph:

> I firmly resolved to use every means in my power, with Divine assistance, to discover a remedy, and, if such efforts failed, to devise efficient methods for alleviating the miseries which accompanied the disease, and for bringing all lepers under the humane as well as the religious influence of the servants of the Gospel of Jesus Christ.[28]

Marsden is modest enough to realize that her grand objective (the discovery of a remedy) may have to be scaled down, but the secondary goals of relieving the lepers' suffering *and* converting them to Christianity still reflect an epic scale. Furthermore, Marsden pledges these goals *after* the journey has been completed, so she knows that the remedy has not been found. Conceivably, then, Marsden still believes when she writes the memoir that she can accomplish the latter goals. More surprising, then, is that alongside and coextensive with Marsden's inferred partnership with Christ and scheme to transform utterly the leper population of Siberia is a corollary rhetoric of humility, and sometimes the interchange between these two positions sounds like a near parody of the 'conflictedness' of women's writing. After a prison visit, she exclaims, 'How unworthy I felt to do this work! But I prayed to God to make me less unworthy. It is a mission that only the noblest, bravest, and purest in the land should do. And I so faulty!'[29] Of course, at every turn the explicit text describes Marsden's noble service, brave resolve and the purity of her dedication; her professions of unworthiness and faultiness therefore suggest either a reflexive imitation of Protestant rhetoric and/or compensation for her heroic self-representation. This dynamic frequently revolves around her changing portrayal of her agency: at times she is only carrying out divine will ('I was only a very helpless tool ... and could do nothing unless God chose to use me for this purpose'),[30] but elsewhere she presents her work as a protracted atonement, which frames her heroism and bravery as the redemptive acts of a sinner. It is this spirit with which she begins the memoir, writing in the preface that 'Readers of the following pages must bear in mind that in the whole world there was no one more unworthy, more full of faults and failings, than I, to undertake this leper work'.[31] In such a context, even her most incredible physical and moral feats may be pitched as compensatory actions rather than grandiose performances.

Her addresses to her readers also operate defensively, as if she anticipates the scepticism that will come to haunt her report and reputation. This editorial self-consciousness occurs more frequently towards the end of the memoir, and statements attesting to the truth of her experience are usually accompanied by references to the supporting documents included in the extensive Appendix to the text. For instance,

> I thought that, as Yakuskt and Viluisk were so many thousands of miles away from all civilization, and so inaccessible, anyone might easily think my account was perhaps only a traveler's tale, and somewhat exaggerated; and this was my reason for having Russian official documents for every statement made.[32]

Elsewhere, she writes that her description of a leper camp 'is but a faint description of what I saw; I have exaggerated nothing, and all I have said can be confirmed by the ispravnick[33] or the priest who live in Viluisk'.[34] Marsden's references to the limitations of her text, like her inclusion of copious testimonies from officials, guides, priests, doctors and sympathetic friends, ironically raise the doubts that she tries to subdue by drawing attention to them. For Monica Anderson in *Women and the Politics of Travel, 1870–1914*, the effect of so many confirming sources is that 'Marsden weakens her own eyewitness accounts by recognizing that they may not be believed. In providing for nonbelief she creates doubt about her reliability as a witness of her own journey.'[35]

The nature of her experiences in Siberia also challenges her powers of representation, as well as the perceived limitations of her readers. While her portraits of the lepers are detailed and vivid (as in her horrifyingly literal account of a leper 'dying by inches'[36]), she alludes to a further, unwritten register of horror:

> I beg the reader to understand that some of the worst details are too repulsive to write about, even for the sake of increasing sympathy on behalf of the lepers. Let it also be understood that all I have said has been verified by others; and, whenever space will permit, I intend quoting from signed documents.[37]

Her sensitivity to the reader's ability to endure a full record of the leper camps finally provides her with an ending to this portion of the text:[38] 'My catalogue of leper miseries, as seen with my own eyes, must now come to an end lest I weary the reader with scenes which, in most of their dreadful aspects, greatly resemble each other'.[39]

Literary and political personas, religious rhetoric and radically contrasting self-representations all make it difficult to extract a very stable picture of Marsden. The object of her journey, too, changes without explanation. The herb is only mentioned twice on the actual journey, and part-way through the memoir she begins to refer to the hospital that she will build. To use Tzevtan Todorov's term for the way that generic formulas furnish interpretive cues, such 'horizons of expectations' are not operable in Marsden's text. As described below, the conflicted role of the Victorian nurse and its governing concept of 'women's work' similarly resists linear or coherent explanation, caught as it is between ideals of sacrifice and professional agency. At the same time, Marsden's growing preoccupation towards the end of the memoir with her own physical breakdown – the irony of the nurse who is herself sick – in fact accords with the rhetorical paradox of the text.

Nursing as a (Suicide) Mission

To understand Marsden's uneven memoir beyond a catch-all nod to its discursive complexity, we need a category that accommodates her movement between 'feeble and faulty' and Christ-like. Throughout the Victorian era, a particular representation of the middle-class nurse drew upon exactly these contrary positions in its representation of 'women's work'. From an ideological point of view, 'women's work' is itself contradictory: the ideal Victorian woman acts selflessly on behalf of others in a purely volitional way, while 'work' smacks of the commercial marketplace and the polluting influences that accompany it.[40] A *Westminster Review* article about nursing from 1888 shows, though inadvertently, the paradox of 'woman's work'. The author calls for improved conditions and higher pay for nurses, advances that would be commensurate with their training and demanding tasks. But in the same article, he participates in the sentimentality that displaces nursing from such professional standards in the first place:

> [Nurses] are the women who carry, wherever they go, an atmosphere of noble labour and unselfish enterprise which brings to this work-a-day world a gleam of the glory to come ... The influence exercised far and wide by a nurse is almost unbounded, and if she be actuated by the fervent love of humanity which urges many women to undertake this work, she can carry everywhere with her a glorious torch to light all upwards towards more sublime and unselfish aims.[41]

The author poses several incongruities in this paean to nurses: 'unselfish enterprise' and 'unselfish aims' follow the same theoretical contradiction as 'women's work', and the description of nurses working on behalf of a 'fervent love of humanity' belies the earlier pledge for better wages. Beyond her repetition of 'women's work', Marsden uses similar colliding descriptions of nursing. Here she appeals to other women to follow her example in Siberia: 'Oh, dear Russian ladies, here is work for you! It is, indeed, women's work. Oh! Let the condition of these poor creatures, guilty though they may be, bring you into this field, "white unto harvest".'[42] In the book of John, the phrase 'white unto harvest' calls upon labourers to reap the harvest;[43] Marsden's address to 'ladies' who will, by way of the Biblical inference, 'labour' thus repeats the ideological paradox of 'woman's work'. On another level, this appeal is undermined by the very memoir that contains it: given the catalogue of horrors that is Marsden's journey, her recruitment scheme seems implausible. The practice of 'nursing the lepers' that underpins Marsden's experience, from her early intentions to find the curative Siberian herb to her eventual contact with them, is itself overdetermined by impossibility. Leprosy was an incurable disease that only became more debilitating and grotesque over time. As Marsden writes, 'the form of their disease is of a very bad nature, and quickly destroys the whole organism, giving the lepers a most awful appearance'.[44] When she prays for 'earnest Christian women to be found, who would be willing to go and nurse the lepers', she implicitly calls on nurses who will accept that the only care they can provide is palliative.[45] The value of their nursing, then, lies in its expression of sacrifice and willing engagement with an alien, 'repulsive' population. But 'willing engagement' minimizes the work, as leprosy nurses and caregivers necessarily endangered themselves.[46] Indeed, leprosy's contagiousness is a prevalent subtext in the testimonials that Marsden includes in her Appendix: the Bishop of Yakutsk mentions the 'frightful contagiousness of the disease', and the President of the Moscow Venerological and Dermatological Society praises her for 'setting aside the possibility of yourself getting the disease among these sufferers'.[47]

Marsden's poor and worsening health constitutes a key topic in the memoir. In the early stages of the trip she chronicles the bruising, cold and exhaustion that accompany sledge travel, but as the journey continues on horseback she 'began to feel the effects of this sort of travelling – in a word, I felt utterly worn out ... the cramp in my body and lower limbs was indescribable'.[48] Finally, after riding through a forest fire ('the most terrible experience of the journey'[49]), '[c]omplete physical exhaustion came at last'.

> So I had to rest, and I began to feel symptoms of an internal malady, which at first alarmed me; and I thought I might have to die there in my little tent, and leave, only just commenced, all the work I wanted to do. But the Master's presence cheered me

> and banished all depression. A day's rest, and then I started again, although in great pain, which, unfortunately, lasted till the end of the journey.[50]

The formula by which Marsden despairs in pain and revives with the thought of God happens more than once, and represents the palliative efficacy of religion rather than medicine – a technique that extends to her nursing.[51] When it comes to her descriptions of her own sickness and weakness, Marsden's awareness of her reader through direct address and acknowledgement signals a need for confirmation and empathy: 'I doubt if any of my readers have ever experienced such utter exhaustion of both mind and body'.[52]

Of course, self-endangerment reifies the saintly nature of her work and her poor health amalgamates extreme bravery and worrisome frailty. Either of these characteristics alone would limit Marsden's heroism and her influence; if she had endured the trip without significant suffering, it would not be convincingly extreme, which her claim to womanly 'feebleness' only underscores. The tension Marsden's text registers between femininity and physical exertion recalls Claire Brock's description in this volume of the female medical student's need to fulfill demanding physical expectations in hospital and retain her 'womanliness' at the same time. Even when Marsden returns to comfortable conditions in Moscow and St Petersburg, she does not fully recover. The Countess Tolstoi, Lady of Honour to the Empress of Russia, provides one of Marsden's numerous testimonials, writing that '[t]he immense difficulties Miss Marsden has overcome have only deepened her zeal for the cause, for which she would willingly give her life, as she has already given her health'.[53]

By its confirmation of her courage and sensitivity, Marsden's physical deterioration activates another narrative about nursing that has a strong precedent in Victorian literature and culture: that of the nurse who is so self-denying that she herself sickens and often dies, effectively 'nursing' herself into the role of the patient. That the best expression of a nurse's morality and dedication is her own death (or its risk) categorically enacts the same conflicted purpose that we see throughout Marsden's memoir on a discursive and rhetorical level. Marsden's representation of or capitulation to illness is analogous to the use of hunger strikes or anorexia nervosa discussed elsewhere in this volume by Sarah Richardson and Susannah Wilson; in each case, the female body is both perpetrator and victim of protest.

Victorian realist fiction, too, provides a steady stream of self-endangering nurses from the 1830s to the 1890s.[54] In Harriet Martineau's *Deerbrook* (1838), heroine Margaret Ibbotsen's unpaid nursing epitomizes the novel's call for civil involvement in a particularly female context. When a typhus epidemic hits the village of Deerbook, Margaret, a young woman who is orphaned and disappointed in love, is asked by a clergyman friend to give her 'time and talents for such services as we gentlemen cannot perform'. Willingly, she goes to the cottage of an infected family where other 'neighbours will not enter'. 'Never before had so squalid [a sight] met Margaret's eyes' as the scene of the suffering family. Her value as a nurse does not lie in her ability to help the sick as three out of her four patients die, but rather in her disregard for her own health amidst the deadly contagion. Where another woman, the Widow Rye, refuses to join Margaret because 'her terror of a sick-room was so extreme', Margaret is propelled by the severity of the risk: 'In a case of such extremity, Margaret had no fears'.[55] Margaret in her selflessness prefigures Marsden's call for 'earnest Christian women ... who would be willing to go and nurse the lepers'.[56]

In Elizabeth Gaskell's *Ruth* (1853), the titular heroine becomes a nurse in part to assuage her guilt over her sexual fall and the consequent illegitimate birth of her son. Thus nursing acts as a form of moral recompense and Ruth, like Marsden, has a special affinity for the most abject and helpless patients.

> She was at the call of all the invalids in town. At first her work lay exclusively among the paupers. At first, too, there was a recoil from many circumstances, which impressed upon her the most fully the physical sufferings of those she tended. But she tried to lose sense of these ... in thinking of the individuals themselves, as separate from their decaying frames ... She allowed herself no nervous haste of movement or touch that should hurt the feelings of the poorest, most friendless creature, who ever lay a victim to disease.[57]

When a typhus epidemic comes to town, 'the nurses belonging to the Infirmary ... shrunk from being drafted into the pestilential fever-ward – when high wages had failed to tempt any to what, in their panic, they considered a certain death'. But Ruth works where these nurses will not: 'I believe I have no fear', she says, and she enters 'right into the very jaws of [the] fierce disease'.[58] Ruth's lack of fear does not mean she evades danger, and in the ultimate sign of her commitment to the sick, she insists upon nursing the infected father of her son. Doing so both kills her and vindicates her character. That the best expression of Ruth's morality is her own death recalls the paradoxical archetype of the witch trial: the innocent drowns and the guilty survives, only to be burnt at the stake.

The iconic experience of Florence Nightingale nearly repeats this dynamic, and though Nightingale avoids death, her reputation as a nurse benefits from the sickness(es) she contacted from her patients. When she returned from the Crimea near death, Nightingale's illness was treated as a natural extension of her work. Victorian critic and historian Mary Poovey writes that England prematurely mourned the death of their national icon and Harriet Martineau, author of *Deerbrook* and prominent writer of non-fiction, readied an obituary that declared Nightingale a model working woman.[59] Marsden, who dedicates *On Sledge and Horseback* to Nightingale, also equates sacrificial nursing to ideal womanhood: 'it goes without saying', she writes, 'that my ideal of an almost perfect Englishwoman is Miss Florence Nightingale; as the queen of nurses to suffering humanity, she stands forth as the embodiments of what a woman can and should be'.[60] If tireless nursing to the point of self-sacrifice makes a woman a queen, then Marsden's own mixture of dejection and grandiosity finds a reasonable prototype.

As much as she feels a 'peculiar thrill'[61] in helping the lepers, Marsden's constant references to her own ill health emphasize her experience as a patient as much as her service as a nurse. At one point she even identifies with the lepers themselves: during a particularly taxing part of her journey, she revives herself with a thought for 'those lepers – they suffered far more than I suffered, and that was the one thought, added to the strength that God supplied, that kept me from collapsing entirely'.[62] At once empathizing with the 'helpless, forsaken' lepers, 'God's worst creatures' and conceiving of a hospital for them at Viluisk, Marsden repeats, albeit in a more sensational fashion, the story of the Victorian nurse who is at once heroic and humble, and so she exemplifies the ideological confusion that is such a prevailing trope in feminist discourse analysis.

Condemned to the Margins

After Siberia, the historical record gives a dismal and cryptic account of Marsden's life. During the fleeting acclaim that she enjoyed following the publication of *On Sledge and Horseback*, she was able to raise a considerable fund towards her leper hospital.[63] In another transformation of her identity, she turns from humble missionary nurse to enterprising capitalist.

The hospital was built, according to Marsden's specific architectural plan, in 1897 and remained open until 1962, a significant lifespan.[64] The beginning of Marsden's troubles in England date from a provocative letter to *The Times* from Alexander Francis, pastor of the St Petersburg British-American church. In the letter, Francis refers to a 'committee of investigation' formed in response to 'a number of serious charges preferred against Miss Marsden by a number of people in England, America, and New Zealand'. Although they were never clarified in *The Times*, historians have discovered that the heart of the complaint was a lesbian relationship Marsden had while nursing in New Zealand. Marsden responded immediately, pleading ignorance; the following day, a letter from Marsden's lawyers threatened a libel suit against Francis.[65] The suit was later dropped, but the public scandal seemed to have taken hold. Well before this, a short article in the *British Medical Journal* (December 1892) accuses Marsden of exaggerating her account of her Siberian journey:

> From a report in a newspaper of a lecture given by Miss Kate Marsden on her visit to Siberia it appears that the lady now admits that she had seen not more than seventy-three lepers, and she stated her belief that there were only between two and three times that number in the whole of the vast Yakutsk district.[66]

Claiming that Marsden 'now admits' how many (or few) lepers she visited contrasts to the memoir, which does not give a specific number. Nevertheless, this is an early example of the cloud of suspicion and accusations of hyperbole that would dog Marsden for the rest of her life. In response to the Francis scandal, she commissioned an authorized and highly sympathetic biography in 1895, but its publication did not have the effect of recovering her name.[67]

Elizabeth Baigent, author of the most complete (and unauthorized) biography of Marsden to date, writes that the original accusation against Marsden by Francis refers to a letter from a woman in New Zealand (where Marsden formerly worked as a nurse) who confessed to a lesbian relationship with Marsden.[68] Details about this purported relationship have not surfaced: it seems that the accusation alone was enough to harm Marsden's reputation. After the campaign against her by Francis, Marsden involved herself in two additional organizations, both of which ended in her premature or fraught withdrawal. She helped found the St Francis Leper Guild in 1895, and converted to Roman Catholicism in order to do so, but was forced to resign in 1899 because of publicity stemming from the original scandal. More than twenty years later, she helped to found the Bexhill Museum, but was again forced to resign when the story of her past was exposed. She published a work in 1921 called *My Mission in Siberia: A Vindication*. As Baigent writes, the book was 'elaborately buttressed' with even more testimonials than the original book, but it did not seem to have much positive influence on either her life or reputation.[69] Marsden lived with a Miss Norris and reportedly suffered very poor health for the rest of her life, dying from senile decay in the Springfield Hospital (earlier the Surrey County Pauper Lunatic Asylum) in 1931. Her public exile, stemming from charges of financial mismanagement and the rumour of lesbianism, seemed finally to overwhelm the work she had undertaken on behalf of the lepers, at least during her lifetime. Her distress for the lepers, as recorded in *On Sledge and Horseback*, takes on a somewhat prophetic meaning in light of her later life: 'Once the community decides that anyone is a leper, he is thus condemned'.[70] By approximately the 1910s, Marsden had indeed transformed permanently from nurse to patient.

Finally, most provocative in the accounts of Marsden's later life is a persistent rumour that she herself had contacted leprosy. Baigent writes that by 1897, Marsden had

> [A]pparently ... been diagnosed with leprosy by a doctor in Honolulu who allegedly obliged her to consult a doctor in Philadelphia. Marsden complained that the false diagnosis obliged her to consult doctors around the world whose fees swallowed her savings ... The stigma following her diagnosis had jeopardized all prospects of employment and a settled life.[71]

Baigent finds it 'fairly clear that she did not have leprosy';[72] but regardless of whether or not Marsden had leprosy or was thought to have leprosy, either possibility replicates the story of the martyred nurse who nurses herself to invalidism or death.

The details of Marsden's later life are scant, and my purpose is not to reconstruct what happened to her as much as to try and understand her perplexing memoir by way of its corollary subjects: Victorian nursing and women's work, leprosy, literary discourse. Together in the memoir and in the fragmented accounts of her later life, these subjects render a picture of Marsden as culturally inassimilable. She is hero and victim, nurse and patient, public servant and liar, and finally, outcast. The symbol that is tempting to adopt, as a paradigm for Marsden's memoir and the controversy that haunted it is its story of origins – leprosy. Again, Marsden's real or professed infection with the disease is immaterial to the way that leprosy's symbolic economy operates: contagiously, incurably and destroying from within, leprosy makes its sufferer into a pariah. In a sensational version of the Victorian nurse whose empathy or exertion renders her as vulnerable as her patients, Marsden's memoir begins with an impossible ambition and over its narrative course as over the course of her own life, self-destructs.

7 CONSTRUCTS OF FEMALE INSANITY AT THE *FIN DE SIÈCLE*: THE LAWN HOSPITAL, LINCOLN, 1882–1902

Katherine Ford

The debate surrounding insanity in the nineteenth century contained a profusion of entangled threads that are still being unpicked by historians today. It was regarded – to borrow a phrase from Elaine Showalter – as a primarily female malady.[1] The construction of insanity as female will be explored here in a twofold investigation, to examine the population of a primarily middle- and upper-class asylum through the voices of the doctors using archival patient records and, in doing so, to reconsider the role that doctors played in the construction of insanity as a female malady in the nineteenth century. This will be achieved through the examination of medical records, completed by medical professionals through direct patient–doctor interaction. Nineteenth-century perceptions of female madness are still clearly traceable in the thinking of English society, due largely to the endurance of popular nineteenth-century fiction featuring mentally unstable females. References to the subject conjure up images of wild or uncontrollable women – Charlotte Brontë's Bertha Rochester or Mary Elizabeth Braddon's Lady Lucy Audley – or the dark, looming presence of the lunatic asylum, which provided a prison for the insane and those mistaken for the mad alike. The most memorable figure of insanity from nineteenth-century fiction is the ostensibly middle- or upper-class female maniac, as seen in little Miss Flyte in Dickens's *Bleak House* (1852–3), Gustave Flaubert's titular *Madame Bovary* (1856) and Catherine Earnshaw in Emily Brontë's *Wuthering Heights* (1847). Conversely, while the Brontës wrote about mentally unstable females, it was a brother who they had (figuratively) locked away in the attic. It has been suggested that while Branwell Brontë is regarded by some modern scholars as a potentially accomplished artist and author,[2] he also suffered from epilepsy,[3] and following an affair with his employer's wife, he slipped into depression, exacerbated by drug and alcohol abuse. The female maniac has been explored thoroughly in literary criticism,[4] but fictional representations of the male maniac is more elusive and significantly feminized, problematically blurring gender boundaries and enforcing the representation of insanity as a female ailment. The veracity of this perception has now been extensively challenged through the literary-historical scholarship of Showalter, Janet Oppenheim and Valerie Pedlar, amongst others. This essay will add to this scholarship using a historical perspective.

The dominant ideologies of the middle classes in the mid-nineteenth century were gender-aligned and centred on the idea of the family. These ideas enforced the idea of separate spheres; confining women to the domestic and allowing men into the public; and imagining women in the traditional mould as vulnerable, mentally weaker and more susceptible to the whims of their emotions.[5] Men, by contrast, were considered superior to women, capable of more physical and mental exertion; this was particularly true in the case of middle-class men who were expected by society to be the self-made men lauded in works such as Samuel Smiles's *Self Help* (1860) and fictionally represented by Dinah Craik's *John Halifax, Gentleman* (1856). Women were expected to submit to their husbands' will and be happy to embody the 'angel in the house' role as domestic homemakers.[6]

The role that doctors played in picturing the insane body as female is particularly complex, with some authors suggesting that doctors are primarily to blame for this conception. In one respect, this is a fair assumption, as doctors were, as middle-class professionals, influenced by the ideologies of their class. As representatives of the middle classes, doctors, therefore, would be expected to maintain the idea that insanity – and the inherent mental weakness it implied – would be more prevalent in the fairer sex. This was, however, not always the case, and here it will be indicated that the role that doctors played in the construction of insanity as a female malady was not so straightforward; instead the perpetuation was part of a wider societal and cultural construct which has since been put under closer scrutiny by historical scholars. The use of the archival material will not only create a picture of the population of one asylum but it will also enable the direct exploration of doctors' words without editing, to investigate whether there is a significant difference in the treatment of the genders.

The matter is further complicated by the status of doctors in society at this time. Medical professionals were fighting for recognition in society and they themselves regarded alienists – asylum doctors and those who studied diseases of the mind – with a certain disdain;[7] even if male madness was prevalent in society, there was a strong chance that any alienist who tried to perpetuate the idea outside of his direct professional environment would face significant hardship, due to the societal pressure upon men as well as women from the dominant middle-class ideologies discussed above. As Oppenheim states, for many, the remuneration for what appears to be a thankless task was so poor that some asylum doctors must have had altruistic motives, choosing the positions 'not simply because some poorly paid jobs were available in asylums, but because they were fascinated with the problems posed by mental illness and were eager to alleviate the suffering of its victims'.[8] Given a lack of resource and personal motivations, the potential for manipulation, concealment or simple ignoring of medical data in popular reports and ideas must be taken into account.

While doctors played a part in the construction of madness as female, the basis of these ideas in a medical context took root long before the nineteenth century in medical writing focusing on the influence of the female reproductive organs, particularly in the type of insanity known as hysteria. Micale states:

> Hysteria is among the oldest described disorders in the history of medicine ... Facts commonly known about the subject [include] that the term *hysteria* traces etymologically to the Greek and Sanskrit words for uterus or womb ... Since ancient times, physicians, philosophers, and natural scientists ... [have] extravagantly theorized female weakness, emotionality and madness.[9]

So, while it is generally understood that the Victorian medical establishment deliberately gendered madness, they were doing so using the tools already set in place by their predecessors and aided by popular media. Moreover, as Oppenheim argues, the 'medical profession ... never attempted to deny the widespread incidence of nervous breakdown among men',[10] yet women were perceived as inherently weaker and therefore more prone to such ailments.

Legitimate alienists were, more than most of the general public, aware of the risks of unlawful confinement, undertaken to perhaps get a problematic spouse or relative out of the way and used possibly to contest legal documents such as wills in 'proving' a family member to be *non compos mentis*. If we consider the links between mental illness and ideas of control – the victim of mental illness could suffer a lack of control or become uncontrollable in their behaviour – then we can see a clear link to ideology of the female, who was not only considered under the sway of her emotions, but was also expected to submit to the will of the dominant males in her life.

That these concerns were felt widely is evidenced by the publication of T. N. Brushfield's lengthy article, 'On Medical Certificates of Insanity', in the *Lancet* in 1880. Brushfield, the first medical superintendent of the Brookwood Asylum in Surrey, contributed this meticulous article detailing the completion of admission certificates in order to provide assistance to medical professionals involved in the committal process, though evidence of its use is uncertain. This article potentially casts the medical profession in a position of protectors to both females and males who were threatened by unscrupulous family members with unlawful confinement, and yet the societal presumption of women as the weaker sex would necessarily present them as more in need of protection. These assumptions, grounded in middle-class values, would naturally apply especially to upper- and middle-class women.

It is relevant, therefore, that there were asylums primarily catering for the upper and middle classes specifically. Accepting mainly or wholly fee-paying patients, these asylums offered a lower doctor-to-patient ratio, enabling the focus on treatment rather than management and often the use of genteel cures such as the promotion of fresh air and exercise. One such establishment was the Lawn Hospital in Lincoln, opened in 1819 as the Lincoln Lunatic Asylum. In 1852, a county lunatic asylum was opened nearby, and by 1880 the patients consisted of fee-paying members primarily of the middle and upper classes; [11] – the Register of Admissions for Pauper Lunatics, which dates from 1845 until 1880, corroborates these asylum demographics.[12] The Lawn was a small establishment, catering for around a hundred patients of both genders, providing them with medical treatment, a routine and recuperation. This was an actual medical asylum, meaning that all the patients admitted during this time period legally required two signed medical admission certificates, although the archives do contain Registers of Voluntary Boarders between 1890 and 1932. The women confined in the Lawn can be taken as representative of their classes, and an awareness of the trappings of middle- and upper-class domestic life was demonstrated in their treatment and surroundings within the asylum. The records will be used in order to examine the proportions of male/female patients and to explore ways in which the medical gaze directly pictured the diseased body through the examination of treatments recorded and through the three medicalized images of patients available in the Lawn records.[13]

Asylums as well as their doctors were frequently viewed with suspicion, a view exploited by writers of fiction at the time. The asylum in *The Woman in White* (1860) is a typical example, where '[even] though doctors and premises seem pleasant enough, the asylum's merciful control is simply a form of imprisonment; it mistakes sanity for madness as easily as it mistakes one person for another'.[14]

The admission papers provide one of the most consistent sources for general information on patients due to their rigid format requesting specific details, and moreover shed light on the knowledge of the admitting doctors. The requirement of two admission certificates each signed by independent doctors was part of a legal system designed to protect people from unlawful imprisonment. They are of historical interest because they provide personal information about the patient, offer a general medical practitioner's perspective of the patient, and allow for the extraction of statistical information, enabling the examination of how the patient was pictured as mentally unfit through the eyes of the doctors. However, while providing a substantial amount of information, the medical value of these certificates is significantly compromised, coming not only through the admitting doctor's gaze – who might not necessarily have any experience of mental health – but moreover via untrained, and often self-interested, witnesses – primarily family members, but also neighbours or community figures – who describe the causes. While, then, the medical data collected from these certificates must be used prudently, it is still a viable source of practical information.

Figure 7.1[15] shows the number of male and female patients admitted between 1882 and 1902. Being a small asylum, the Lawn accepted less than thirty-five patients in any one year over this period. Overall, the number of females is higher than the number of males, but not markedly so and this graph indicates that there was not a particularly consistent pattern of admission. For nine of the twenty-one years covered, the number of female patients accepted is equal to or less than the male patients and in only three – 1883, 1897 and 1899 – are the numbers of female patients submitted significantly higher[16] than male patients. The asylum was not, then, inundated with female patients, though the numbers were marginally higher than male patients overall. Over this time period 45 per cent of patients admitted were male and 55 per cent were female. While it is true that the Lawn Hospital cannot be taken as a typical asylum of its time, it is indicative of care for a certain class of patient.

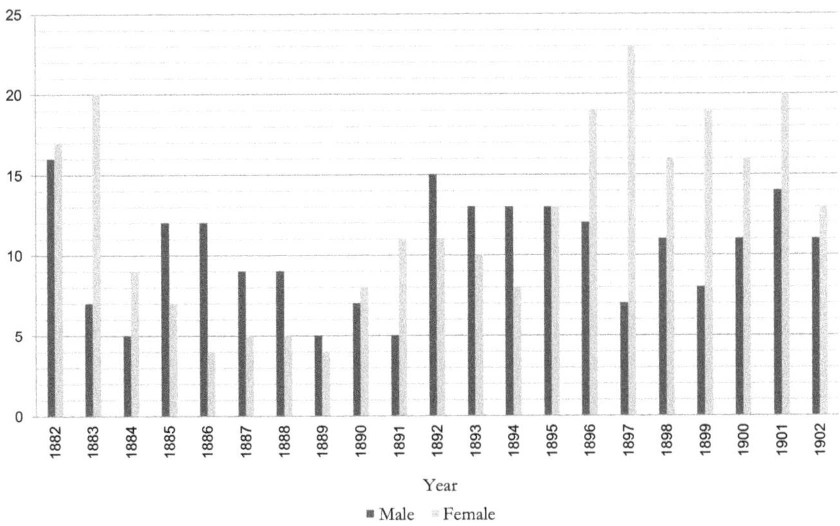

Figure 7.1: Patients admitted by gender, 1882–1902, the Lawn Hospital, Lincoln. Data taken from Lawn Hospital Admission Papers, 1882–1902.

The class of the female patients can be seen in the listing of occupation on the admission certificates.[17] While some are evidently working class, the three largest groups are those who have no occupation. Firstly, there are those who are described under the occupation of wife, widow or daughter. Secondly, there is a group of women of independent means or 'gentlewomen' – a very Victorian perspective of middle-class women's work – who were expected to be managing their households, thereby fulfilling the 'angel in the house' ideal. Thirdly, there is a section of inmates who work in a profession, either in domestic service – primarily ladies' maids or general housekeepers, suggesting a closeness between themselves and a person of the upper or middle classes and thus explaining their admission here rather than the County Asylum – or those involved in schooling within the home, a means of living necessitating a fairly high level of education and placing its practitioners above the working classes, but which would not make an individual personally well-off. All the roles of female patients were placed squarely in the domestic sphere and were typically female roles.

Gender roles are apparent in the patient section on the admission certificates, where the person recommending the committing establishes his or her relationship with the patient. In almost every case it is a family member, unless no close familial tie existed. This is a reflection of the idea of madness as a domestic concern, one which was to be kept, as much as possible, within the family. It is unsurprising that patients were usually committed by family members as it was with them that they spent most of their time, and if there was an indication of a behavioural shift towards violence – noted generally as a yes/no response to the 'dangerous to others and in what way' option on the admission certificate – on the part of the patient those within the domestic sphere were most at risk. Husbands and wives, parents and children all played a part, but employers were also, in certain situations, willing to step in. Young women were often brought in by their mothers rather than by other family members, and son-in-laws would frequently step in if their wife's mother became mentally unstable. The links between those who did the committing and the patient were frequently decided by age. Mothers and fathers were common in the case of younger patients, but as the patients got older, the family members varied, and children, nephews and nieces assumed the role of the committee. That family members were the main committers enforces the idea that mental troubles were considered a personal and domestic issue. This was also emphasized as, in the majority of cases, family members contributed the secondary evidence for the admission certificate. That mental illness was confined to the domestic is a reflection of the wider social structure of the late Victorian period, with the family at its centre, and moreover, the role that the family played in confining patients ensured that this structure was perpetuated.

Figure 7.2[18] shows the gender relation between the patient and those committing them. The levels of males committed, both by females and other males remains primarily below ten, as does the number of females committed by other females, with the erratic nature of the graph indicating the fluctuating number of patients committed as a whole. The number of females committed by males appears to make substantial leaps at points, but this also must be considered alongside the overall increase and decline in the numbers admitted to the asylum yearly, as indicated in Figure 7.1. Referring back, we see that the asylum had an overall increase in the number of female patients taken in over this period.

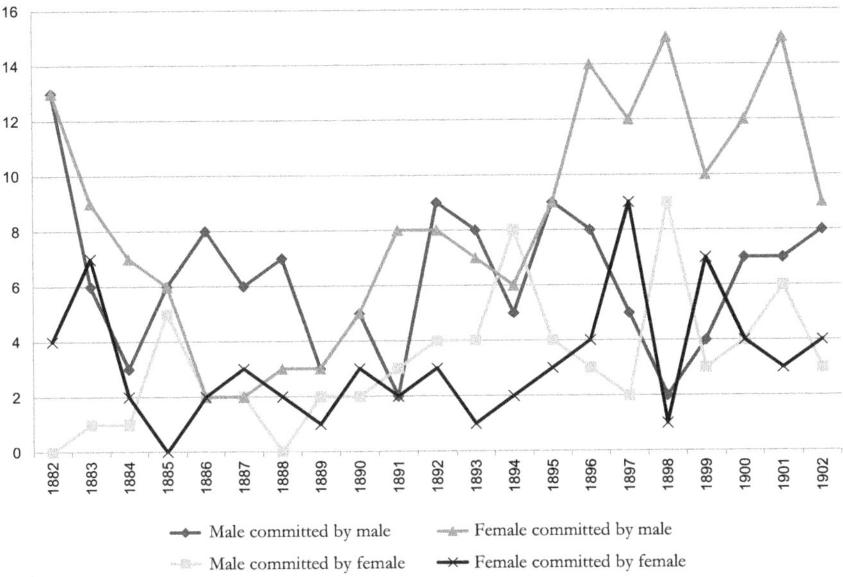

Figure 7.2: Committees: gender comparison, the Lawn Hospital, Lincoln. Data taken from Lawn Hospital Admission Papers, 1882–1902.

That the majority of committers were male is symptomatic of the patriarchal potency endemic in the nineteenth century, but the graph also crucially shows that males were not the sole wielders of committing power; females also played a significant role in the process. Taking into consideration that the upsurge in female patients comes at the end of the 1890s, when women were increasing their political power and making themselves heard, this is more likely an anomalous reflection of the overall rise in patient numbers of the Lawn, as it gained in popularity or capacity, rather than indicative of a cultural change or a backlash against the female desire to regain their power.

As previously mentioned, the medical section on the admissions certificate was completed by a medical practitioner who was not required to have any special expertise in mental health. Folsom noted in 1881 that '[if] we look over the list of alleged causes of mental disease in the reports of our insane asylums, we find that they vary according to the theories of the medical officers recording them'.[19] Figure 7.3[20] illustrates the primary reasons cited on the forms between 1882 and 1902, and the sheer volume of 'unknown' responses indicates the lack of knowledge of many medical professionals when faced with the need to diagnose something that they did not understand, or at least did not have enough confidence to diagnose. The reasons themselves are not necessarily accurate, as the writer frequently cites the trigger for the outward manifestation of the attack.

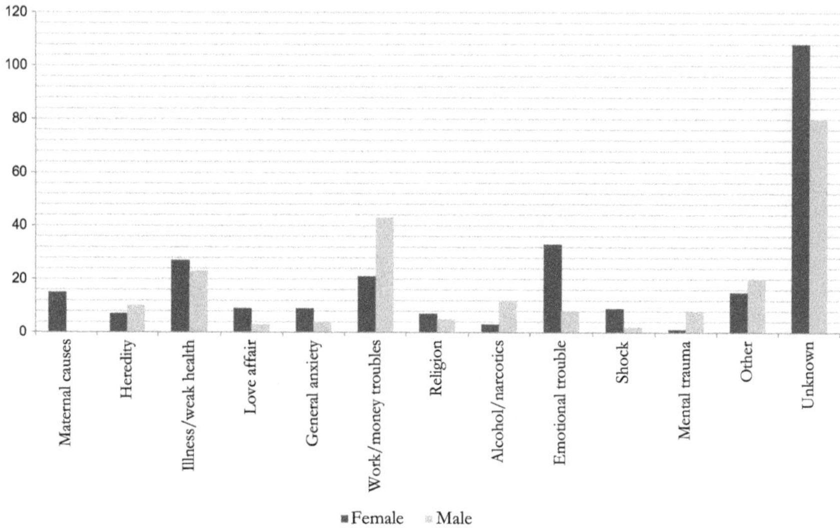

Figure 7.3: Cause of insanity, the Lawn Hospital, Lincoln. Data taken from Lawn Hospital Admission Papers, 1882–1902.

Still, the data indicates that doctors were nearly 15 per cent more likely to cite 'unknown' as a cause in cases of female mental breakdown. The citation of 'unknown' as a cause in 41 per cent of female cases over this period, while potentially demonstrating a lack of information on the part of the attending physician, can also be read as an implication of the perceived vulnerability of women to mental breakdown for no apparent reason. Moreover, it indicates the female's supposed lack of control over her own mental well-being, an idea that is emphasized when considered alongside other female-dominated causes for insanity revealed in the graph. These relate to emotions and weak health, implying that proneness to mental collapse is encoded into women's bodies, naturally linked to their vulnerable nature. Given that the information here is taken from either an admitting doctor or witness testimony, these reasons are filtered through common perceptions of insanity – those even doctors were susceptible to. Women were more likely to fall prey to emotional trouble, general anxiety and maternal causes. It is significant, however, that males are not so very far behind in cases of weak health, and perhaps surprisingly, women were also admitted due to work and money troubles. There were also a small proportion of men admitted due to love affairs, traditionally associated with female insanity. Notably there was a separate section on the admission certificate to state whether there was any history of insanity in the family, and the admitting doctor did not always make a connection between the two. Failure to do so is potentially indicative of contradicting conclusions, not all mutually exclusive: firstly, that the doctor completing the certificate did not make the connection between insanity in the family line and the patient; secondly, that the doctor did not believe the connection pertinent in this particular case or thirdly, the reason for admission could be confidently attributed to a separate cause. However, while indicative of the medical gaze, the cause for the attack was not necessarily framed by the doctor as the evidence indicates it was more likely to be taken from the testimony of the witnesses who gave statements for the certification.[21]

Once within the confines of the asylum, conditions varied widely, depending on the size and the type of asylum, the way they were funded and the staff that ran it on a daily basis, particularly the medical superintendent. The Lawn was a private asylum but it also aimed to be a charitable institution.[22] The patient fees were designed to cover upkeep, food, activities and the salaries of the staff, but it was not run for profit. Despite the range of fees there is no apparent evidence of a strong class divide within the asylum, although those paying higher fees maintained a higher standard of living. The general rate for a patient in October 1883 was 30 shillings per week, or £78 per year, but one patient was recorded as paying £158 per year, and the other fees paid ranged from £130 per year down to around £60 per year,[23] demonstrative of the range of middle- and upper-class patients at the Lawn.

The domesticity of the asylum assisted in picturing the environment as female. This was, after all, the age of the 'angel in the house' and home, as already mentioned, was central to the ideology of the middle classes. Food, as befitting a homely milieu, was clearly an important part of structure in the hospital. Patients were observed closely at mealtimes, especially if they ate little or nothing; details of their diet were presented in their case notes and patients were given suppositories or fed milk and eggs if they suffered from weak stomachs or were feeling unwell.[24] Oppenheim notes that diet was important to asylum doctors because, among other reasons, 'medical wisdom claimed that nervous exhaustion was frequently aggravated, if not occasioned, by a delicate stomach or painful indigestion hindering the transmission of nutriments to weakened nerves'.[25] Symptoms of this kind moreover encouraged the feminization of the mad person, as it associated them with a delicate, weakened form. Modern psychological theories suggest that in cases of disorders such as anorexia nervosa, sufferers refuse food, as it is something they feel they have a measure of control over, and this could certainly apply to patients within the Lawn as well.[26] Anorexia as a disorder and particularly as a form of control is explored by Susannah Wilson elsewhere in this collection.[27] The control of diet is an example of the moral management of patients; ensuring that they were fit and healthy in their bodies would, it was hoped, enable them to maintain better command under mental duress. It is not possible to tell whether it is primarily male or female patients who are not eating properly, though it seems from the case notes to be a spread across both genders and all ages. Interestingly, lack of appetite is traditionally associated with lovesick females who are typically melancholic in character, but the case notes here illustrate that lack of eating was, at least in recorded cases, connected with paranoia, as in the case of Thomas Gauntley, who was noted in the case notes as having 'delusions that his wife poisons his food and ... [refuses] food in consequence'.[28]

The activities available to inmates were observed and recorded by the Commissioners in Lunacy as they completed their biannual inspections. Activities were promoted that were considered healthy and suitable for ladies and gentlemen of the middle and upper classes, promoting moral and physical health. Patients were encouraged to be out of bed and to take plenty of fresh air and exercise, ideas which were perpetuated in wider society, as Alexandra Lewis notes in her essay on *Villette* elsewhere in this collection: Brontë shows awareness that 'physical stasis curtails, or even contaminates, mental life'.[29] Reading and playing the piano were promoted for the ladies and the purchase of a new billiard table was encouraged for the male ward as '[the] present table is small, poor and in bad order'.[30] Once patients were considered to be improving, they were encouraged to write letters. These activities were all considered part of the moral treatment that alienists provided for those in their care. The inmates were also, where possible, taken on day trips and to the seaside for a change of air, for medical purposes and also to assist in maintaining contact with the outside world. Both the male and female pursuits were considered to be activities that conjured up images of domestic felicity – however unlikely such situations were in the patients' homes – aiming to put the patients at ease and contributed to an atmosphere in the hope 'that homelike mental institutions would tame and domesticate madness and bring it into the sphere of rationality'.[31] These theories were more specifically aimed at females, as the home was their expected environment – particularly given their social status – and societal assumptions offered no place safer than home.

Within the asylum, balls and dances were held for the patients, attended by members of the local community, which fostered a feeling of participation in normal life and indicated that the asylum was part of the wider community. A comment in the case notes indicates that showing interest in one's surroundings was a sign of improvement and thus a step further on the path to recovery. Balls and other events were a way of piquing the interest of otherwise distracted patients. When the weather was good, everyone was expected to be outside unless confined through illness, thus associating exercise and fresh air with health. The outdoor activities the patients pursued were also indicative of their class, as was the divide between the pursuits of the genders. The men, if able, would take part in sporting games, such as croquet, and the ladies would generally walk or sit in the garden.[32] The patients could also work in the grounds or the laundry, assisting with the upkeep of the asylum if they wished to, indicative of the middle-class association between health and hard work. Contrary to popular belief, doctors also allowed patients a degree of free movement, and did not regard treatment within an asylum to be of indefinite duration. That the Lawn patients were allowed two levels of temporary release – at the discretion of the administrators – concurs with this point. Patients could be granted parole to go to church and out for walks around the city, presumably when it was considered that they were trustworthy enough to do so (and more or less guaranteed to return).

Within asylums, the medical treatment that patients received varied, though there is no difference in medical treatment received by males and females; in the Lawn Hospital records, there is very little information regarding the treatments used for the conditions which placed them in the asylum in the first place. The Medical Journals chronicle general illnesses, complaints and injuries that occurred in daily life. The case notes available refer most frequently to chloral, designed to encourage sleep and to stop fits; potassium bromide, used to control fits primarily in epileptic patients; and castor oil and tincture rhei to aid bowel movement. In some serious cases, patient behaviour was monitored and recorded closely and medical treatments cited on these sheets are the administration of either castor oil or enemas. Treatment for fits is often simply documented as 'medicine', which presumably either refers to the use of potassium bromide to control fits, or to chloral, in which case the patient is usually recorded as falling asleep, although the form of treatment and resulting effects could potentially be omitted from the case notes.[33] The nineteenth century witnessed the birth of psychiatry, and hospitals like the Lawn provided a recuperative environment for those suffering from 'shattered nerves', which in turn gave the doctors an opportunity to observe and to try and cure using new methods. Oppenheim notes that this point in history was a launching point for the use of psychotherapeutics, but that doctors were unwilling to treat only the patient's minds,[34] hence the emphasis on diet and physical exercise.

The case notes, while not providing extensive information on patient treatment, do provide the possibility of hearing the patients speak for themselves, which is rare, '[given] the limited number of accounts scripted by patients themselves'.[35] They are, it is true, filtered through the medical gaze of the attending physician who recorded the notes, but they regularly record the patients' words apparently verbatim, and indicate the careful watch that the doctors kept on the patients. Furthermore, while many examples of patient communications are now surfacing, those suffering from delusions, or in the depths of depression or mania, could not or would not wish to document their thoughts and feelings. Letters are in existence, and through these it is possible to view accounts of the patients' thoughts and experiences first hand; however, in some cases the words are so confused that they are of limited use to historians. Case books are, within the Lawn's records, all that remain of these interactions and they tell us about the doctors as well as the patients. It must be noted that it is difficult to ascertain the voice of the speaker; while this could be construed positively, presenting the speaker as impartial, it also means that it is easy to forget that there is an intermediary between the words coming from the patient and as they appear to the modern reader in the form of the recording physician. Thus, it must be remembered that the patients' voices are subject to 'editing' via the physician's decision of what is of significance to record. The notes are generally brief, implying limited time for one-to-one patient–doctor interactions but they include a good deal of detail concerning patient behaviour, eating habits and sleep patterns.

The archives include a volume of photographs dated *c.* 1899, a collection of images which enable us to view the patients. The purpose of these photographs – whether they were taken for physiognomical study or other medical uses – is unknown. Showalter notes that some asylum doctors regarded photography as a medical tool:

> Dr Hugh Welch Diamond ... physician to the female department at the Surrey Asylum ... argued that ... it was salutary to have this reminder of personal appearance, and to have the natural feminine vanity, dulled by disease, stimulated by a photographic portrait.[36]

While it is unclear whether patients were shown the portraits taken within the asylum – indeed, it seems unlikely, given their setting and the somewhat sickly appearance of some of the patients, they would stimulate the 'feminine vanity' – there are loose images marked as taken by professional portrait artists within the volume which suggest that Diamond's idea was implemented. The layout of the photographs contained within the volume suggests that a general copy was kept for the use of the doctors or administrative purposes and though Diamond also argued for the value of photographs for physiognomical study, there is no evidence in the medical records to indicate that this was undertaken. Diamond's characterization of vanity as naturally feminine and as a motivator for healing implies shallowness on the part of female mental weakness, one which can at least partially be remedied by a reminder of their 'healthy' appearance and by suggesting this as an aid to recovery superficiality is implied as inherent in the feminine psyche, and vanity is outright stated.

Some photographs, like Figure 7.4,[37] were evidently taken after a patient's recovery, this one bearing what appears to be a warm inscription to Dr Russell on the reverse, stating 'For Dear Dr. Russell With Celia Emily Place's love and all good wishes for future health and Happiness'.[38] Such tokens suggest that the work that asylum doctors did was not always underappreciated. There is no information on this particular patient available, but the sincerity with which the message is worded implies gratitude on the part of the writer, the warmth comes from the message and places her not as a patient but as an individual. The woman in the photograph is sitting in a position of power – her hand controls the cart and she sits upright, erect, compared to the man next to her. Even if we alter the inherent assumption made here – if we take the male to be the patient, a relative for whom our writer is expressing gratitude – then the female still proves to be the most powerful figure in the image, and a woman may well have had to take control in the case of her relative's well-being, as indicated in Figure 7.2.

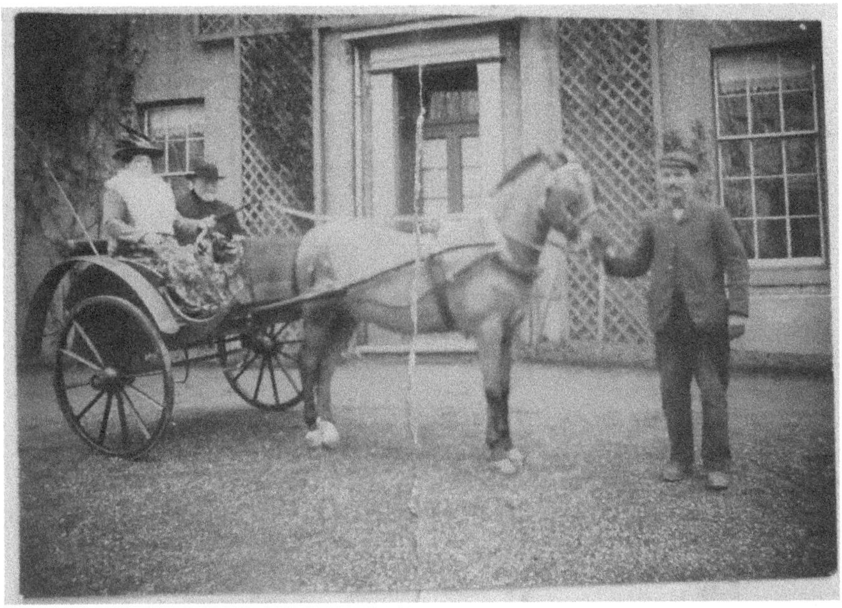

Figure 7.4: Memento photograph to Dr Russell from Celia Emily Place, Lawn Hospital Volume of Photographs, *c.* 1899, loose image. Reproduced courtesy of the Lincolnshire County Council Archives.

There appear to only be a handful of photographs within the volume which can be regarded as tokens; the majority appear to be portrait-style photographs taken within the asylum gardens. There are also, nonetheless, three images in particular which display the patient in a medical way. Figure 7.5[39] shows a set of four photographs displaying a severe case of skin discolouration on the legs of a male patient. Medically, it is unclear what has caused this, although it is possible that it is self-inflicted or of some kind of ill health not necessarily connected to the patient's mental state, given that another patient admitted in 1880 was noted as having '[a] number of bright patches on his chest and abdomen'[40] along with very weak health due to his refusal to eat. The most telling element of this image is that in the two images on the right, there is a nurse visible and another hand keeping the patient's legs apart, his own arms being drawn up against the body. Although clearly a male, the patient is depersonalized with his head out of frame and the nurse in the photograph looking towards the condition rather than at the patient's face. The image is, moreover, desexualized by the close wrapping of the groin and the only reason it is possible to really tell that this is a male patient is by referring to the name in the case notes. Combined with this, the arms are drawn up protectively towards the body, heightening the sense of vulnerability of the patient and thus effeminizing the figure. The patient here is vulnerable as well as depersonalized; the male-on-male medical gaze is clinical and is concerned directly with the skin condition itself rather than the patient. The image is clearly a medical image taken to document a specific medical condition.

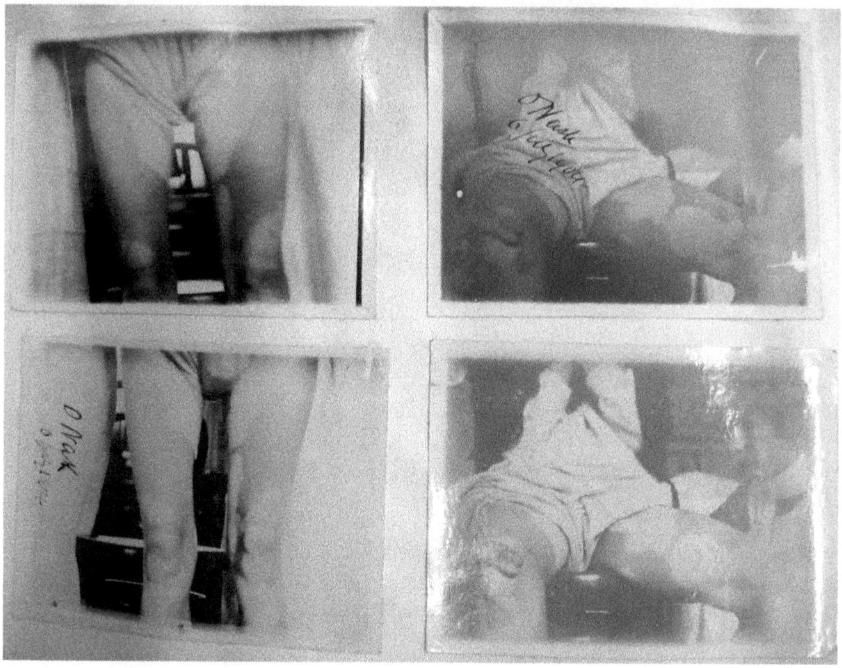

Figure 7.5: Untitled medical image, Lawn Hospital Volume of Photographs, *c.* 1899. Reproduced courtesy of the Lincolnshire County Council Archives.

Figure 7.6,[41] however, is less clear in its purpose, and appears to be of unknown afflictions. Without the benefit of a name or any accompanying case notes, it is difficult to ascertain the cause of these raised welts on the patient. As in the previous image, it is of a male patient and focuses on the patient's body with the head out of frame. The view of the camera in relation to the subject emphasizes the feeling of vulnerability, as in the last image, appearing to gaze down on the body, and the positioning of the body itself indicates that the legs and arms may well have been held in place in order to capture the image, although it is likely that had the patient been struggling fiercely the shoulders would have also been held. The patient is almost entirely naked, with the shirt lifted up and tucked around the chin, adding to the sense of exposure. While there is no explanation for this image either with it or in the case notes, it is self-evidently taken for medical purposes. Again, regardless of whether these injuries were self-inflicted, caused by another inmate or symptomatic of a condition, there is a clear reason for this photograph and the record that it provides.

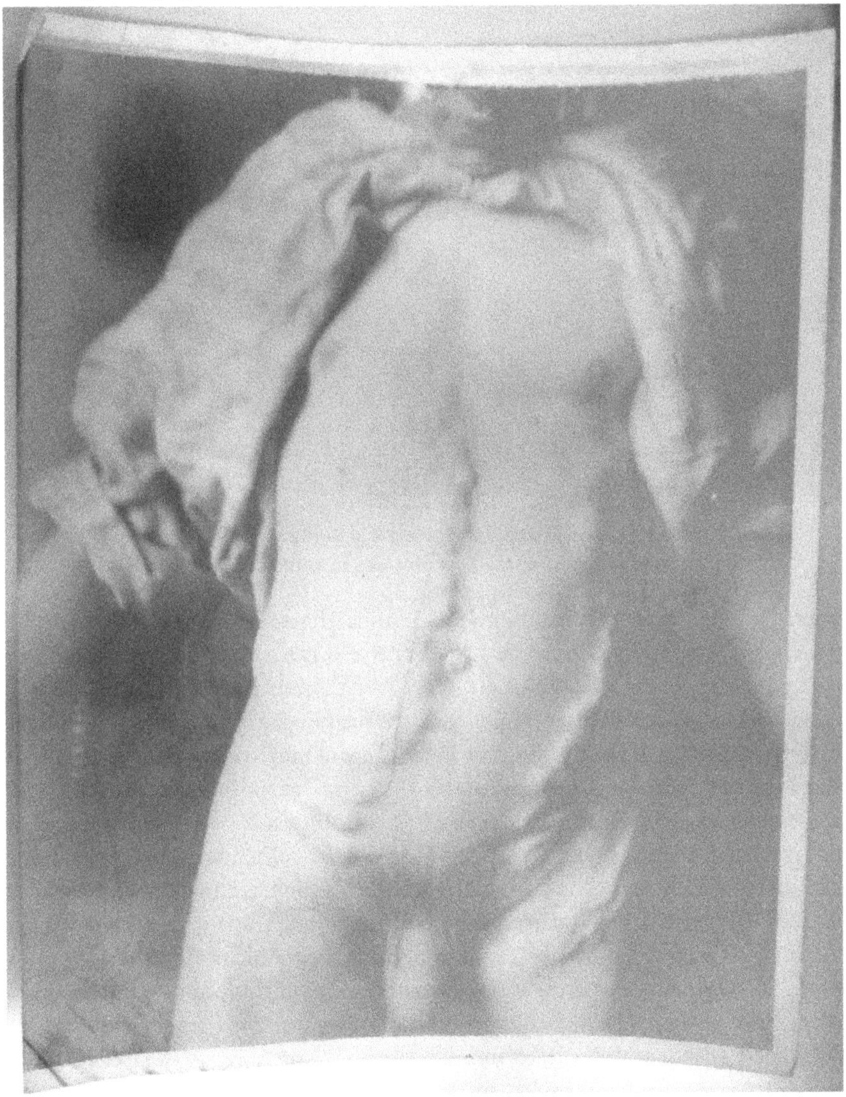

Figure 7.6: Untitled medical image, Lawn Hospital Volume of Photographs, *c*. 1899. Reproduced courtesy of the Lincolnshire County Council Archives.

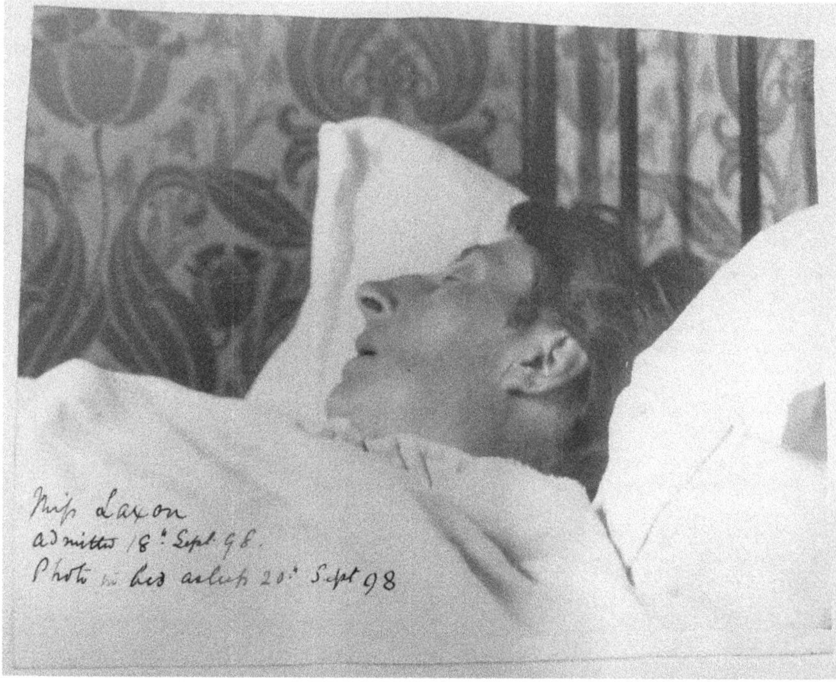

Figure 7.7: Marion Laxon asleep, Lawn Hospital Volume of Photographs, *c.* 1899. Reproduced courtesy of the Lincolnshire County Council Archives.

Figure 7.7[42] is even more ambiguous. Unlike the previous photographs, the patient's face is firmly within the frame, and this is the only surviving medicalized photograph of a female patient. The patient's body is covered completely by bedclothes and even if this were not the case, the photograph centres on her face, with the majority of the body out of shot. There are no marks or anything out of the ordinary visible on the patient's face. The sense of exposure here is in the presentation of the subject: the patient sleeping is emblematic of the vulnerability of not just this patient, but of *all* patients. However, as vulnerability was considered a quintessentially feminine characteristic, images such as this reinforce ideas of feminine subjectivity and surrender – be it to mental illness, or men – within madness. The image is fortunately labelled so it is possible to find the case notes for the patient, but once these are found, the reason for this photograph becomes even more obscure. The labelling on the photograph itself reads 'Miss Laxon: Admitted 18th Sept. 98, photo in bed asleep 20th sept. 98'.[43] The image, then, was taken two days after she was admitted. There is a reference to her hair being very scanty and the possibility of skin disease, but the image here documents no evidence of any such conditions. When compared with the other two images, this feels intensely subjective; we know details of who the patient is, but not why the image was captured. When we delve into the case notes, it becomes apparent that her case was not particularly out of the ordinary; she was committed by her father after suffering from delusions and suicidal tendencies and was in the hospital for eight months, finally being discharged as recovered after being treated for a thyroid problem, the treatment for this beginning some three months after her arrival at the hospital. The differences between these three photographs are quite stark, demonstrating the different ways in which the medical gaze focused on male and female bodies. This indicates that doctors were directly influenced in their picturing of male and female medical conditions. The male conditions are clearly documented by these photographs; however, when we explore the case notes of Marion Laxon, there was no recorded reason why this photograph was taken, and no immediately obvious evidence in the photograph itself. In the male photographs it is the exposure of the body itself that gives the vulnerability, but in the female photograph the body is not exposed; rather, it is in the position of the patient and the attitude of the medical gaze watching her. The depersonalization in the male medical images means that the patients are successfully divorced from their condition, able to exist as both men and patients as we do not know who the men are, whereas the shot of Marion Laxon is an intensely personal one, and she is inseparable from her medicalized state. In her essay on anorexia, Wilson argues that the removal of the face from images or photography in death heightens the voyeurism implicit in the photographs;[44] the patient is an inactive participant, and this reading can be applied to the photographs of the male patients also. However, while her face is within the frame, the voyeurism in the photograph of the female patient is also palpable. While not dead, the passive nature of her condition removes her direct participation. The constructions of male and female medical conditions in these images, taken by or under direction from the medical staff, personalize the female patient's infirmity but separate that of the male patients.

The disparity in focus between male and female patients offers a preliminary indication, underscored by recent scholarship on perceptions and realities between male and female insanity in the nineteenth century, of the differing way in which the primarily male medical gaze regarded male and female medical states. While there are, admittedly, only three cases available here for comparison, the obvious medical conditions documented in the images of the male patients contrast with the medicalized situation of the female patient with no apparent symptoms documented in the photograph.

The stigma associated with the asylum must surely have stemmed in part from the apparent finality of the decision. Yet, looking at the Removal, Death and Discharge records for 1880–1902 at the Lawn, patients clearly did leave asylums. Realistically, patients could generally expect a stay of less than five years in the Lawn, and between 1880 and 1902, 161 male and 192 female patients were discharged with only 30 males and 25 females marked as not improved, while the rest were either noted to be recovered or relieved. The reasons for release in the cases where no improvement has been made are not always stated, but it was usually at the behest of a family member.

Patients could be transferred to another asylum without any improvement – this is proportionally rare, occurring twenty-two times in the cases of male patients and twenty-four times in the cases of females. Transfers primarily occurred in the first five years of the patient's committal. This makes it clear that in most cases the decision to move a person was made early and principally for financial reasons, although there are instances of later moves for the purpose of being closer to relations or when the financial toll began to show in cases of long-term committal. The similarity in number to those discharged as not improved could indicate that the latter group was taken home where provisions had been made for their care. There was no significant difference in the number of male and female patients who recovered or were transferred, although female patients were nearly a third more likely to be discharged as relieved than male patients – which links back to the higher level of 'unknown' verdicts on the admission certificates. If there was uncertainty as to what triggered the mental breakdown of the female, it could well mean that the asylum doctors believed that another attack was a possibility. Again, this places the female's mental health out of their own power; they were relieved – or in modern terms, in remission – but not necessarily cured. The proportion between those who recovered, however, was not so different, with eighty-four male and ninety-seven female patients recovered. The similar recovery and discharge rates between males and females show that insanity as a primarily female malady was in part a construct, as there is not a significant enough difference in number to merit the gendering of the illness as prominently as was the case.

Duration of stay in the asylum was regarded, as aforementioned, as an indefinite sentence. Perhaps this was because the stays in fiction seemed so unlimited (though they rarely were, even in seemingly impossible situations) and also because sensationalized media accounts of trials resulting in lifetime incarceration in criminal asylums were rife. The data in Figure 7.8[45] challenges this, showing a comparison of duration of stay for male and female patients. Both groups were almost equally likely to be discharged in the first three years of their stay, and half of those patients spending less than three years in the asylum were discharged in under a year. Neither men nor women were likely to spend more time in the Lawn than the other; each had their share of hopeless cases. For both genders, the longer spent in an asylum meant that there was a higher chance of dying within its walls, but this was more likely because there was no one or no way to care for them at home. Interestingly, of the patients who did die in the Lawn, many had not been in the asylum for an extended period of time.

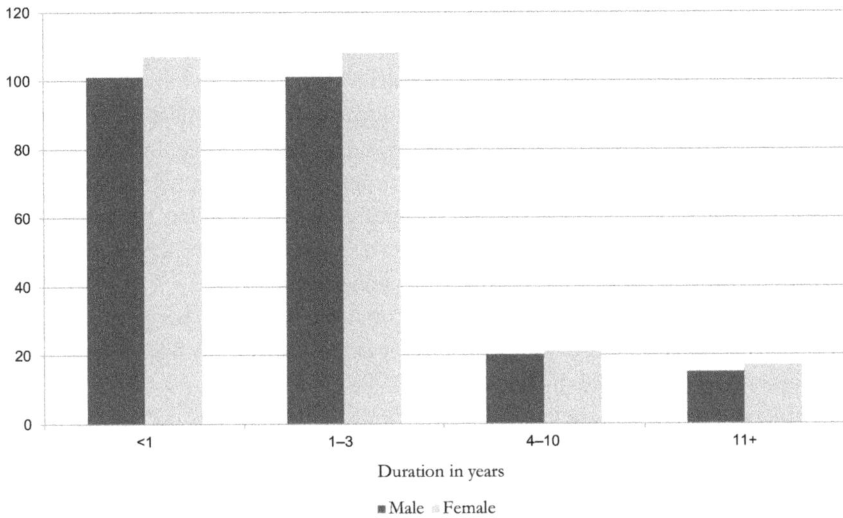

Figure 7.8: Duration of stay, the Lawn Hospital, Lincoln. Data taken from Registers of Removals, Discharges and Deaths 1873–90, 1890–95 and 1895–1906.

Realistically, while patients did die in asylums, these cases were more likely to be committed in the final years of their illness when the patient could no longer be cared for. Especially in instances of General Paralysis, mental decline was likely to worsen as the disease progressed and their final years were when they were most likely to be committed, and they would, therefore, die less than five years into their confinement. Those who died from General Paralysis generally died between their mid-thirties and late forties, although there were two patients in the Lawn between 1880 and 1902 that survived until sixty and seventy. Male patient deaths peaked around age forty in the Lawn, around a third of them caused by General Paralysis, though a higher number were attributed simply to brain disease. Female deaths, on the other hand, peaked in the seventies. That women died so much later than men was not a reflection on their likelihood of being discharged – as the data has shown – rather, it was symptomatic of their sex, as women lived longer than men and also reflected on the causes of death. Once the terminal stages of General Paralysis were reached, men could not hope to live long, and died younger. The presence of older women in asylums perpetuates the idea that women were victims of long-term incarceration, but the truth is, like their male counterparts, many of them were only taken in for a short length of time, since as both genders got older they weakened and thus became more prone to mental disturbances. Some stayed for an extensive period, it is true, but as men were likely to die at a younger age, this left a majority of older women in the asylum population. In terms of duration of stay, the results show clearly that the majority of patients who were discharged were most likely to leave in the first five years of their confinement, and even the majority of those who died or were transferred spent five years or less in the asylum. The amount of time passed in an asylum is in inverse proportion to the likelihood of release; a significant deviation from popular conceptions. For example, in Wilkie Collins's *The Woman in White*, Laura Fairlie's incarceration appears to be indefinite; there is no mention of any possibility of release for her – she has no option but escape. Popular representations such as this were based in cultural perceptions of the time, and Collins exploits this fear for dramatic effect.

The Lawn Hospital records show, then, that the difference between the male and the female population of the asylum were not always so disparate. Given, however, that at this time the dominant middle-class ideology portrayed women as vulnerable and attempted to keep them firmly within the domestic sphere, evidence seen here demonstrates how the ideological assumptions were still applied to these women, within and without the asylum. The women confined in the Lawn were representative of their classes, and the perceptions of their class filtered the gaze that they were under, from admission through to discharge. The doctors who confined them were handicapped by their lack of knowledge and the perceptions of the familial witnesses. Once inside the asylum, they were still treated as ladies and the medical treatment they underwent was the same as that of male patients. While doctors could not escape the societal perceptions of the female maniac, this did not mean that they were responsible for this perspective; though they were products of their class and society they still aimed to treat male and female patients alike, reflected here in the similar discharge rates. However, the conclusion reached in the discussion of the photographic images indicates that they did not always succeed in this. That women lived longer accounts for the perception that women were likely to be kept in asylums longer, as the average age of death for females was much higher than that of males within the asylum – but in the majority of these cases they were simply committed later in life.

The predominantly male medical gaze picturing the male and female bodies here does reflect the inability of doctors to escape from the perceptions of femininity. The images discussed here indicate a preoccupation with conditions but the careful depersonalization of the male images and the ambiguity of rationale behind the female photograph imply a carefulness to separate the male from the condition, a care which is not taken in the case of Marion Laxon. While doctors were products of their social environment, this did not mean that they medically treated their male and female patients differently; however, their perceptions coloured their judgement in diagnosing, documenting and describing patient conditions. The picture of the lifelong imprisoned female madwoman was imposed by society, not by the doctors, but they played a role in perpetuating the idea which has, in part thanks to literary interpretations, endured ever since.

8 THE FITNESS OF THE FEMALE MEDICAL STUDENT, 1895–1910

Claire Brock

In 1905, former Honorary Secretary of the London School of Medicine for Women (LSMW), Isabel Thorne, published a small account which celebrated thirty years of the institution. While this was intended primarily as an historical narrative describing the foundation of the School, it also contained portraits of a few illustrious and talented alumni, some of whom had died tragically pursuing their goal. The final paragraphs of the *Sketch* were directed firmly at the 'successive generation of students', those lucky ones for whom the road had 'been cleared and the way made easy' and whose only burden was not the individual struggle borne bravely by their predecessors but a collective weight of social and professional expectation.[1] For the early twentieth-century female medical student, carrying 'on the traditions handed down to them', following 'in the footsteps' of the great names meant exhibiting both skilfulness 'in the practice of her profession, but also [as] an example to all other women for purity of mind and large heartedness'.[2] Isabel Thorne concluded the *Sketch* with a flawless portrait of the 'ideal qualities' of the medical woman:

> She should be wise and sympathetic with a clear, logical mind, much common-sense, good judgment, tact and acquaintance with human nature, able to inspire her patients with confidence. She is brought into close contact with so many of her fellow creatures, has so much varied experience of trying situations, that she requires not only a profound knowledge of medicine and surgery, but a firm grasp of the principles underlying them and the faculty of applying what she knows to suitable cases. She must be unselfish with a great capacity for taking pains. If she takes up surgery much practical skill is needed. She sees so much of the sorrows of life that her heart is often wrung by the griefs of her patients who depend upon her for counsel and comfort in their troubles. She must be able to face responsibilities, for the issues of life and death are often in her hands, and much depends upon her judgment; good health, too, is a most important condition. A medical woman should possess a combination of all that is best in womanhood. Her profession gives her sphere of action for the exertion of the highest qualities. We look to present and future generations of medical students to justify the hard struggles of the pioneers of the movement and to show

> their appreciation of the efforts which have been made to secure to women liberty to be trained for the medical and surgical treatment of their own sex.[3]

To embody all the requisite characteristics of a successful female doctor, the medical student needed mental, moral and physical fitness for her chosen career, while retaining every facet of her womanliness. It is hardly surprising that some students found their years at medical school and the demands of 'community life' 'strenuous'.[4] For the *fin-de-siècle* and early twentieth-century female medical student, stamina was all. Pressure to succeed, without breaking down in mind, morals or body, was inculcated from their first day at the LSMW by the pioneering generation, who had battled for acceptance by society and the profession itself and desired to maintain a formidable reputation for uprightness and strength.

This essay will explore the tensions between such expectations and experience of life as a female medical student through a case study of the LSMW, its student publications and records, over a key fifteen-year period in its history. The institution was founded in 1874 by medical women and their supporters because of their frustration over repeated attempts to block them from qualification through other means. The first and, therefore, 'Mother School of all British Medical Women' to which, as Isabel Thorne put it, every female medical student should be 'indebted', was linked to the Royal Free Hospital for clinical instruction in 1877 and a year later the University of London, when it began to award its degrees to women.[5] In 1895, the students of the LSMW started their own magazine, prefaced with the School's motto, 'Work is as it is done', inextricably associating hard graft with accomplishment and success. Reviewing its first issue, the *British Medical Journal* (*BMJ*) concluded that while the 'contents were of the usual character' for a student-led production, the LSMW *Magazine* possessed an even tone, blending '*utile* with *dulce* in a satisfactory manner'.[6] In two years, the *Magazine* had 300 subscribers among students and graduates alike. This had increased to 409 by 1908; 259 of these were qualified.[7] The majority of material for the *Magazine* came from students at the School or Hospital, but the editor was usually already in practice, as were some of the correspondents, who were encouraged to write in about their medical life after graduation.[8] As Laura Kelly has recently remarked, the magazine is a curiously under-researched, but fruitful, source of information about medical student life.[9] Such publications also allow 'largely absent or silent consumers' to speak.[10] The ways in which the students of the second generation of medical women shaped their collective identity against their predecessors through this publishing venture, as well as how they pictured themselves, will give an insight into how the female medical student of the late nineteenth and early twentieth century managed her studies and attempted to maintain a healthy equilibrium in the face of private, public and professional strains.

'The Much-Abused "Lady Medical"'[11]

When women had first agitated to join the medical profession in the mid-nineteenth century, their fitness to practise was an argument employed both by supporters and detractors.[12] Women's access to higher education was being hotly debated at this point, rendering female medical students doubly suspicious because of their desire to profit professionally from their tertiary training. In 1870, the *Lancet* argued that

> women are neither physically nor morally qualified for many of the onerous, important, and confident duties of the general practitioner; nor capable of the prolonged exertions, or severe exposures to all kinds of weathers which a professional life entails; nor capable of keeping the social secrets of patients, which are often dearer than life, and are second only to the claims of justice; nor ought they be able to give instruction on many points of worldly wisdom which often serve to save many from temptation, or even to reclaim them from actual sin or impending ruin.[13]

Physically, mentally and morally weak, naïve, gossipy and inexperienced in the ways of the world, women were simply not capable of coping with the harsh realities of everyday medical life nor maintaining high professional standards. Medicine and women were effectively antithetical. On the contrary, for supporters, peculiarly female qualities made women especially suitable for the medical profession. As an anonymous pamphleteer noted, merit, rather than sex, should dictate who could practise:

> All women may not be fit for such work. *But all men are not fit for it.* Many women will lack the necessary amount of nerve; but *many men lack it also.* In difficulty and danger women have great presence of mind. They are often calm and collected where men are unhinged and unbalanced, and incapable of exertion. Women have more tenderness and more patience, and they must necessarily understand many female ailments better than men. They will always have one great advantage over male practitioners – female patients will be more unreserved in their communications to them.[14]

For this writer, femaleness was eminently desirable in a medical practitioner. Such attributes ultimately saved lives, which was surely the *raison d'être* of the profession.

While such debates reduced in intensity as more women qualified successfully, doubts about women's capabilities resurfaced occasionally when isolated incidents were generalized, by press and profession alike, to argue for female medical unfitness. In 1903, the suicide of Sophia Frances Hickman, a recent, multiple prize-winning graduate of the LSMW, who had just begun a locum position at the Royal Free Hospital, sparked a lengthy correspondence in newspapers and periodicals about women's inability to cope with the pressures of the job. Despite Miss Hickman's personal robustness (she was 5ft 9in and powerfully built), fondness for long walks and intellectual strength, which were drawn upon frequently in reports, speculation was rife as to what had caused her to take her own life. When she disappeared without explanation in August 1903, she was pronounced by her family to be in the 'very best health both mental and physical'.[15] Before the discovery of Miss Hickman's badly decomposed body in Richmond Park two months later, little by little, her reputation was eroded by the (predominantly lay) press until it was concluded that even an outstanding student, possessed of an abundance of mental and physical stamina, could be harbouring doubts as to her abilities and concealing a congenital heart condition.[16] For Sophia Hickman's contemporaries and for current students at the LSMW, the 'calamity' which had 'befallen' them all was reported with 'difficulty' and in solemn tones.[17] As the *BMJ* kindly noted, with recognition of the strenuous nature of the profession for men and women alike, Sophia Frances Hickman's tragic end did not imply all women were incapable of carrying out their duties: 'to suggest that all women are unfit to practise medicine because one of their weaker sisters has fallen by the way and failed in her self-appointed task is to draw a false conclusion from the particular to the general'.[18] Some of the students reading this notice would surely not have felt comforted by the acknowledgement of the number of medical practitioners of either sex who had not been able to fulfil their responsibilities. When even the strongest of students had succumbed, weakness was clearly very much to be feared.

'The Life of a Medical Student is a Trying One'[19]

In spite of the *BMJ*'s defence of the woman doctor after the Hickman case, women were in a different position to men when they applied to become students. While many more girls had been educated to a higher standard than ever before, they had not always studied the sciences in any depth and many struggled with even preliminary examinations. Although female students saw the funny side of tutors mocking them for their 'small knowledge' of such 'masculine' subjects as physics and chemistry, 'reaching the standard' required was a genuine concern.[20] Social pressures meant that they had to be careful where and with whom they chose to live or to associate while studying, especially those in London. And, of course, they were often subject to the disapproval of friends and family, even as late as the 1910s, as Octavia Wilberforce, who studied at the LSMW between 1913 and 1920, would so painfully illustrate.[21] The different advice for male and female students in Charles Bell Keetley's popular *The Student's Guide to the Medical Profession* (1878/1885) is particularly pertinent here. While many student textbooks focused on study or upon specific parts of the medical curriculum, Bell Keetley offered the prospective students and their parents a glimpse into the lifestyle of medicine. Co-founder and later Dean of the LSMW and the first woman doctor to qualify in Britain, Elizabeth Garrett

Anderson, contributed a chapter on female education to the *Student's Guide*. From the outset, Garrett Anderson makes it clear that women will be more 'closely scrutinised' than men and can, as such, 'less easily afford to be second-rate': 'The standard of professional attainment will be higher than that expected in the case of the ordinary male'.[22] Educational achievement for a female student needed to be superlative. However stern her advice, Garrett Anderson counselled women not to be swayed by anyone else: 'I would beg female students of medicine not to be discouraged either by the magnitude of the work to which they have put their hands, or by the disapproval of many of their friends and acquaintance'.[23] The strength needed to defy familial expectation must be coupled with physical stamina. Both Bell Keetley and Garrett Anderson draw attention to the potentially healthy lifestyle of the medical practitioner, but do so in very different ways. The former suggests that those of 'delicate' constitution could actually 'gain strength during their medical studies', in spite of the professional side-effects of exposure to infection or night work. 'Dissipation', however, is the chief moral failing of the medical student, which, in turn, leads to the undermining of physical health.[24] While the male medical student dissipates his health away, the female works away hers. As Garrett Anderson makes clear, female medical students do not 'break down' frequently; when they do, it is solely through overwork and lack of rest. Even the student who, for want of funds or simply boasting, notes that she can live upon *6d.* a day, becomes a 'complete wreck' through a combination of insufficient nutrition and 'hard work'. '[G]ood food, and plenty of it, long nights, and thorough holidays' should lead to a 'very healthy life', according to Elizabeth Garrett Anderson.[25] Female medical students needed to be well-balanced, maintaining an equilibrium between work (although always at the highest level) and rest (taking every advantage of their rare time at leisure).

Health was also a concern of an 1895 *BMJ* article on 'The Cost of Medical Education'. Costs, the periodical advised, were not simply financial; although an estimated bill of between £587 and £734 for five years of study in London might have caused both prospective parents and students to blanch. The changing attitude towards the medical student in the nineteenth century, the transformation from the badly-behaved dilettante to the disciplined professional, is very much in evidence in the *BMJ* advice.[26] Any 'slip', whether that be intellectual or because of ill health, could only prolong the course; those insufficiently committed due to personal distaste for medical work, family reasons or lack of funds were 'absolutely wast[ing]' their time, but also their prospects, so 'peculiarly special' was the profession.[27] In order to avoid a breakdown in constitution, 'considerable' outdoor exercise was advised and, presumably due to the solitary nature of study, team sports such as boating, cricket, tennis and football were heartily recommended. While, warns the *BMJ*, this side of life can occasionally be 'overdone', it is 'absolutely essential': the medical profession were prone, by their very occupation, to depression and early death.[28] Unlike Bell Keetley's suggestion that medical life could bring health to even the most sickly, the *BMJ* warns of the essentially solitary nature of practical student work in dissecting rooms and laboratories. Therefore, spare time should not be spent alone, but in the company of others in vigorous exercise. Identifying oneself as part of a team would encourage discipline and responsibility, as well as contributing to the formation of a professional outlook. The difference in opinion between guide and periodical can be explained due to the latter's typically *fin-de-siècle* concentration on the importance of raising and maintaining national fitness.[29] Medical predisposition to an unhealthy state of mind and body finally leads the *BMJ* to conclude that the 'athletic side of education is really more necessary for the medical than for any other class of student'.[30] In order for medical students to be fit for their chosen profession, their bodies, as well as their minds, needed to be fully and regularly exercised.

While the *BMJ* worries about the 'unhealthy' atmosphere of medical and surgical spaces, such as laboratories or operating theatres, late nineteenth- and early twentieth-century female medical students were repeatedly portrayed as thriving on such noxious fumes. In an 1897 *Ludgate* article on 'How Women Doctors are Made', former student of the LSMW, Arabella Kenealy, told a very different tale of the professional space:

> From early morning till late evening we occupied the backless stools on either side the leaden tables, following the course of muscles, veins and blood-vessels with studious knives. Beside us lay our open books, which we from time to time consulted; sometimes we asked questions of one another, or listened to the admonitions of our demonstrator. But for the most part we were a silent, intent group. Legends we heard of dissecting-room vagaries of masculine students, but they failed to inspire us.[31]

The female students here work independently, but never solitarily. Indeed, what is noticeable here is the camaraderie and harmony between the women; the silence is companionable rather than sinister. While their 'masculine' counterparts are inconsistent and unpredictable, female medical students are neither impressed, infected nor affected by tales of such behaviour. Instead, they proceed solidly and methodically, inspired only by their work. The dissecting room was, of course, one of the environments which especially shocked opponents of medical women, who believed femininity and dissection were fundamentally incompatible.[32] That Kenealy and her colleagues refuse to imagine the horrors points to their devotion to serious medical studies and their professionalism; both of which are, as Kenealy implies, over and above that of 'masculine' students.

In the October 1902 edition of the LSMW *Magazine*, 'A Lover of Truth' wrote to the editor with an anecdote about the misdirected over-zealousness of a male medical graduate after a hansom cab accident. While this 'Lady Medical Student' was indeed run over, no 'important limbs' had been amputated and no 'complications' had ensued; her 'Shocking Injuries' and 'critical condition' were press fabrications.[33] Indeed, but for a couple of 'minute bruises', the supposedly 'hapless patient' was uninjured. Taken to St George's Hospital, the 'Lover of Truth' detailed her actual experience, which differed considerably from the harrowing tale told by the press. What is fascinating about this letter is the way in which the writer views her male contemporary. Swooping in to examine his 'prey', this 'very babe in years' makes 'lightning' diagnoses, which range from a tuberculous knee to a fractured patella and 'ankylosed' joint: '"that is to say, you will never be able to bend it", he explained kindly'. The 'Lover of Truth' listens patiently to the young resident's conjectures, dismissing each conclusion with a statement which proves his inaccuracy, all the while silently mocking his 'professional manner', which was 'worthy of a Harley Street specialist'. Unable to come to any firm decision, the perplexed man offers his patient a bed, which she refuses and instead asks to go 'home' to the 'London Royal Free Hospital School of Medicine for Women'. This leads to a fleet departure of the embarrassed doctor, recommending, as he leaves, an extract of opium for the patient's knee. While the patient is happy to extol the way in which the nurses, the porter and the police handled her accident and the general splendour of the hospital itself, her treatment by the young male resident passes without comment. Although he attempts to impress with his learning, his inability to examine the patient, his overly lofty, unsupported diagnoses and his lack of interest in hearing an account of her accident marks his behaviour as unprofessional. Such an attitude, argues 'A Lover of Truth', would never characterize a 'Royal Free' student, who would 'seldom, if ever' guess at a condition without thorough examination. As the Royal Free only trained female students from the LSMW, 'A Lover of Truth' jocularly, though vehemently, defends the thorough, careful education of medical women. May well the resident flee in shame, she implies, at the mention of the School and its training hospital.

Late nineteenth- and early twentieth-century female medical students were inculcated from the start of their training about uprightness in the face of the more difficult aspects of their career. Revealing any 'feminine' emotion was strictly condemned. As Arabella Kenealy remarked, while many might 'shudder' over their first operation and seek a 'reviving breath of air' in the courtyard afterwards, the self-control of the female medical student was legendary: 'We, however, punctiliously stopped short of fainting – for it was a point of honour with us to beat the record of our masculine counterpart who distinguishes himself notably in this direction'.[34] From the outset of women's campaign to enter medicine, they had been attacked both for a lack of strength and an inability to conquer either physical or emotional distress. Here, however, Kenealy suggests that women simply 'shudder', but do not give way or break down, regaining composure swiftly and completely. Their male colleagues, in contrast, actually 'distinguish' themselves through their weakness. Those who ran the LSMW were also keen to stress female *sang froid* to the curious. Interest in the LSMW and the female medical student grew in the 1890s as the School expanded. Indeed, the academic year 1895–6 saw sixty-four new students enter; this would be the largest cohort until the jump in numbers encouraged by the beginning of the Great War.[35] Press coverage also increased, especially after the summer of 1898, when the Prince and Princess of Wales opened the new laboratories at the School and correspondingly signalled their approval of the study of medicine for women. A reporter for the weekly illustrated women's periodical *Madame* indicates the level of public curiosity in an article entitled 'The London School of Medicine for Women'. Upon arrival, the young porter greets the journalist with a 'familiar grin' when an interview is requested: '"Many Press representatives been here lately?" "'Undreds of 'em", replied the youth'. As well as encountering and subsequently photographing 'students at work', the reporter remarks upon 'the look of rapt intensity', the 'absorbing interest in their study and intention to succeed'. Ambition and determination are evident in the faces of the students. Miss Douie, the School Secretary, confirms the steadiness and commitment of the students, whom, she stresses, carry out 'precisely' the same training and examinations as their male counterparts. '"I may say"', notes Miss Douie, they "do remarkably well in their examinations, some gaining marked distinction"'.[36] It is hardly surprising that the students are more than capable of remaining 'quite still', without wavering in their dedication, while they are captured intent upon their studies. Only one regards the photographer, slightly quizzical about the proceedings (Figure 8.1).

The tenacity of the female medical student was also something which was frequently mentioned in press articles about the LSMW. As the *London Argus* remarked, upon the occasion of the visit of the Prince and Princess of Wales in 1898, 'few women give up the study of medicine' and the combination of 'sympathy' and 'skill' has endeared the medical woman, once qualified, to her patients.[37] Elizabeth Garrett Anderson, then Dean of the LSMW, had proffered similar comments to the House of Lords Select Committee on Metropolitan Hospitals in 1891.[38] Quizzed extensively about medical women and their capabilities, Garrett Anderson defends her students against assumptions of inadequacy or any marked difference from their male colleagues. At this point, she notes, while only one woman, Mrs Scharlieb, had passed the MD (London) degree, 'only one per cent of the men who enter the medical profession' achieve this advanced accolade. Given the fact that the only woman who had entered so far had passed, Garrett Anderson allowed the statistics to speak for themselves.

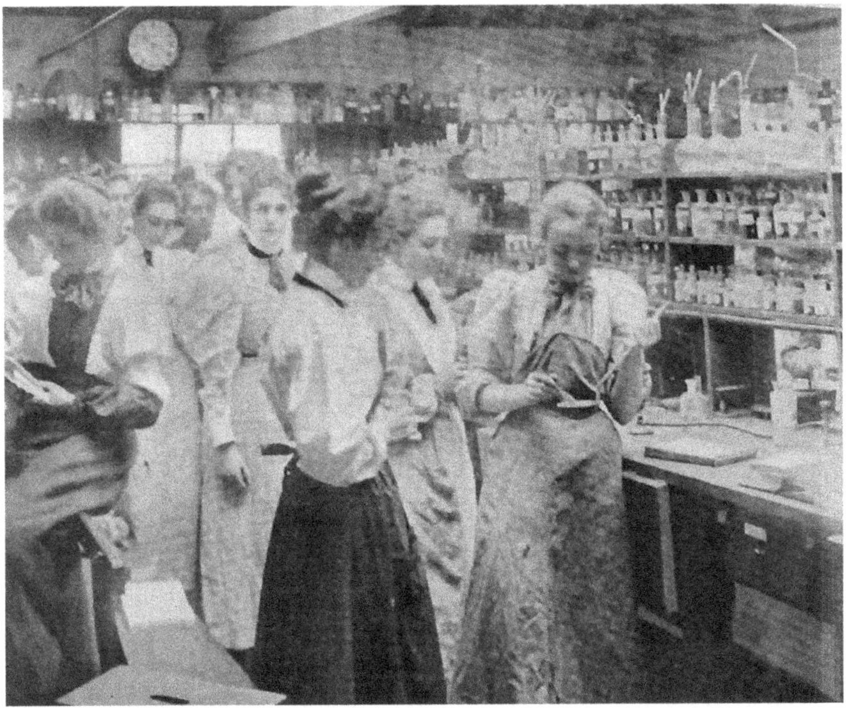

Figure 8.1: 'The London School of Medicine: The Chemical Laboratory', *Madame* (June 1898), pp. 782–4, on p. 782. Reproduced courtesy of the Royal Free Hospital Archive Centre, Royal Free London NHS Foundation Trust.

Nor were there concessions for 'femaleness'; all studies were 'exactly' as at any other medical school. In response to a question from the Earl of Arran about the evident desire of women to enter the 'lucrative profession', the Dean agreed and remarked that 'failure' was not a word she would associate with medical women. They would certainly not succumb easily. Only 'continued' and, therefore, prolonged and incapacitating, ill health or the lack of suitable qualities in the first place would put a stop to studies. Women were far from constitutionally unsound to practise medicine. Probing further, Earl Cathcart enquired if 'women had strength enough of wrist to [perform surgery]?' Garrett Anderson's monosyllabic affirmative swiftly dismisses any concern about bodily strength. The Earl of Arran closes proceedings with a question directed precisely at the student experience: 'Would your experience lead you to think that it takes your lady students longer to get used to the terrible sights and scenes in the operating theatre than it would men students?' Garrett Anderson responds by denying she has much knowledge of male students, but she can be positive in her understanding of the mind of the female medical student:

> I do not know that I have ever heard of any of our women fainting; I have heard of men fainting occasionally; but I daresay it takes both of them a little time to get used to it. I have never known of a woman leaving off the study of medicine because she found it too dreadful. They soon become deeply interested in it.

For all the supposed 'horrors' of medical study, Garrett Anderson reveals the stamina of female students, who, unlike their male counterparts, remain upright, alert and engaged throughout.

Garrett Anderson's boast was certainly not an idle one. Examining the statistics of entrances and exits from the LSMW, very few students leave courses for reasons other than marriage, ill health or death. Indeed, between the 1894–5 and the 1910–11 academic years, only an average of 8.44 per cent of students withdraw from their studies. Across the same period, an average of 74.3 per cent of total entrants eventually qualify. Withdrawals reached their nadir in 1906–7, when a third of entrants withdrew, but there are two academic years, 1897–8 and 1905–6, when none leave.[39] It is interesting that when numbers fall dramatically in comparison to previous years, the press quickly pick up upon and attack the School for its exits or the LSMW moves to defend itself against the possibility of such accusations. In 1894, twenty years after the opening of the medical school, May Dickinson Berry, a former student, wrote to the *Lancet* to defend the 14 per cent defection rate over the past two decades.[40] Against the quoted 8 per cent of withdrawals out of a total of 1,000 students at the all-male Bart's, the numbers look high, but Dickinson Berry suggests that demands upon women are far higher as far as family is concerned. Ironically, while Dickinson Berry utilizes femaleness here to excuse those unable to finish the course, she concludes with a warning that this should not imply that women lack 'steadfastness'. Indeed, given their multiple social roles, it might be said that they embody it.

Examining more closely student files, alongside the *Register of Students*, not every withdrawal has a reason beside it, but the staff were clearly keen to keep a record of departures given the ways in which the career of the female medical student was closely monitored by press and profession alike. Between 1894 and 1911, there are forty-four withdrawals and fifteen reasons given for the student's inability to complete the course. There are two deaths, three illnesses and one marriage. While this latter student does not have any further information about her future, one who marries in 1913, 'M. B. L.', writes with the deepest regret to announce her nuptials, devastated at losing work enjoyed 'so much', which had only become 'more and more interesting'.[41] Marriage was not always an escape for the less able; medicine was not given up without regret. Other reasons include taking up another course, such as physiology or chemistry, or a desire to study elsewhere. Two re-enter at a later date, seven and eight years after initially starting their course, while another later qualifies as a doctor. All reveal genuine and longstanding commitment to their calling, despite a lengthy period of intervention between the beginning and end of their medical studies. The final few are more complex. One, 'M. E. M.' is 'prevented from continuing' her course, presumably due to financial constraints, although no further information is available. 'C. B.' suffered from deafness, which was causing her difficulties in her studies, while 'F. K.' is 'dismissed' in 1910–11. A read-through of her quite lengthy file reveals her youth (she was only seventeen when she began her course) and consistent and exasperating failure in examinations (which were attributed, kindly, to her age).[42]

'M. V. E.' is perhaps the most curious case of withdrawal from the LSMW, as her departure had nothing to do with either academic or physical failings, but rather the more shady area of 'moral' shortcomings. Noted as a new student in the Spring Term of 1893, 'M. V. E.' was still at the LSMW in 1902, when she was 'dismissed'. In similar fashion to 'F. K.' she possesses an unusually bulging file of correspondence both by and about her, although the latter predominates. The first reference to any impropriety on the part of 'M. V. E.' is to be found in the Minutes of a 'Special' Meeting held by the Council of the LSMW in May 1901. Under the section entitled 'Dismissal of Student', the Dean, Elizabeth Garrett Anderson, makes a report, which concludes, after a 'full investigati[on]', that the name of Miss 'M. V. E.' should be removed from the list of students. Garrett Anderson's letter is included in the Minutes and reads as follows:

> I am sorry to have to report that it has seemed to me to be necessary to dismiss a student.
>
> I became aware that she was making very serious charges against a fellow student. I called upon the accuser, heard her story, and was told by her the names of various people who could, she believed, confirm it. I saw all these separately, and could not get a scrap of confirmation. I saw the accused who absolutely denied the statements made against her. I saw a near relative who told me that similar accusations had before been made by the accuser. I have since come upon a second accusation, of a kindred character, made by the same student against another fellow student which I believe from the circumstances must be absolutely false. I have also in my possession an apology from the same student for a third calumny which she started some years ago and from which she in the end gave a written apology. I look upon the accuser as mentally unsound, but she is very plausible and dangerous. I saw her a second time and told her I did not believe her charges and I then suspended her. After careful further enquiry, and seeing her parents, I have told her that her name is no longer on the list of the school or Hospital students.[43]

While this does not leave any indication as to what precisely 'M. V. E.' had done, it is clear that deliberate falsehood is involved and repeated attempts to besmirch the reputation of others on the part of 'M. V. E.'. At no point is the word 'immoral' behaviour used and yet 'M. V. E.' launched an action to claim damages from the School for ruining her name. An extract from the *Daily Telegraph* of 13 June 1902 is included in the 'M. V. E.' file, which details the case brought against the School. Although the incident 'promised to be of some importance', the matter was cleared before an action could begin. The LSMW 'wished it to be stated that they had made no reflections whatever upon the moral character of [Miss E]'; the comment was 'publicly made' because of the nature of the case. An unsigned handwritten statement, also within the 'M. V. E.' file, acknowledges the information given in the *Telegraph* report, but adds a remark about the 'considerable expense' to which the Council were put and that they had never made an 'accusation of immoral conduct'. Fascinatingly, within less than a month of this agreement, 'M. V. E.' wrote the briefest of letters, dated 9 July 1902: 'I ask that my name may be restored to the List of Students in connection with the LRFHSMW'. Hardly surprisingly, although the Council do meet to discuss her 'readmission', after 'full consider[ation]' they reply just as succinctly that they have decided 'not to accede to it'. There is no further comment from 'M. V. E.'.

Leaving 'the Sheltering Wing'[44]

The treatment of the 'M. V. E.' case illustrates the increasing use of discipline in medical schools, keen to attract the best and most committed students, in the late nineteenth and early twentieth century.[45] 'M. V. E.' reflected badly upon the LSMW both because of her own actions and her accusations about the dubious behaviour of a number of fellow students, implying a laxness about the scrupulousness of entry standards, in spite of the reputation the School was keen to uphold. This lack of fit between the actual attitudes of female youth and the ideal student so cherished by the older generation of medical women clearly shook the LSMW's belief in its processes. That 'M. V. E.' had entered the School nine years before and had not learned from her experience meant she certainly could not return to her studies. Her very presence would remind the staff of their own mistakes in harbouring 'M. V. E.' for so long. With such expectations from their teaching staff, students at the LSMW had an enormous reputation to maintain. When Elizabeth Garrett Anderson resigned as Dean less than a year after the 'M. V. E.' debacle, she left, as the School *Magazine* reported, having imprinted on the students her 'incapacity to tolerate the second-rate'.[46] Female medical students must not compromise in 'carry[ing] on her traditions to the utmost of [their] power', noted 'An Old Student', who wanted to see only an unbroken chain of achievement and success, a 'pattern' of consistency handed down to future generations.

The LSMW *Magazine* reveals how aware the students were of their need to perpetuate and keep up appearances of an ideal medical woman, but also a desire to reshape the designated mould into which they were to be poured. There are few non-medical illustrations in the magazine throughout the fifteen-year period covered by this essay, but when they do appear they are always satirical line drawings in the manner of *Punch* and its ilk, poking fun at the profession or patients. One particular illustrated piece from January 1905, 'Some Notes on the Studentology of the Neighbourhood of Hunter Street and Gray's Inn Road', mocks the different species of female student to be found at the LSMW. While this etymological study notes that there are types into which most students can be grouped, it will not accept that there is one homogenous female medical student (see Figures 8.2–8.4). The 'Studentology' divides the LSMW students into six separate kinds, representing variety, but also levels of mental and physical development: the *Vermiformix Bibliomania*; the *Aesculapia Athletica*; the *Aesculapia Aquatica*; the *Vainessa Itinera*; the *Antifeminina Inormata*; and the *Dressara*. Hearty, sporty and energetic, *Aesculapia*, who belong to the order 'Leapandhoptera', are hardy, outdoor specimens, fit and strong. In contrast to the *Aesculapia*, the *Bibliomania* is of the order *Neurotica* and can be characterized by her pale, hunched, small, inert body and enormous head with bulging eyes, the result, no doubt, of spending all her time indoors, surrounded by books. Though she consumes voraciously, rumours concerning her transformation into a beautiful creature are much exaggerated. Remaining at this larvae stage, the *Bibliomania* can eat her way through much source material, but, with all her efforts, only a fraction of it is assimilated. The *Antifeminina* or stick insect can be placed among the Manlikidae. She is masculine and bespectacled, with close-cropped hair and a thin, tall body. Her outer coverings are as dull and boring as her demeanour, but serve as a repellent to potential predators. The *Vainessa* is the opposite of the *Antifeminina*: she is flighty and bright only in her external appearance. She rarely haunts the area of the Medical School during working hours and can more frequently be found flitting about in the West End of the city, only returning after dark. Lightness, brightness and noise attract the *Vainessa*, unlike the *Bibliomania*, who despises all three. Finally, the most advanced, but also the cruellest: the *Dressara*. Unlike the other forms, this one groups together and can be found at all times and in all seasons. Positioned in the distinctive order of the Cutyewuptera, this species causes fear and terror to most humans, upon whose 'broken surfaces' they fasten themselves with speed and delight.[47]

Students to be found in the 'Neighbourhood of Hunter Street and Gray's Inn Road' are a composite mixture of all the stereotypical assumptions about women pursuing medicine or higher education in general: dowdy, underdeveloped, mannish, bookish and neurotic. And yet they also thrive in outdoor pursuits, socialize widely, play as hard as they work and actually enjoy their studies. They can also be beautiful and interested in fashion and fashionable pursuits. Time and again in the *Magazine* of the LSMW it is possible to witness female medical students having fun with the images expected of them by profession and public alike. Reports of external visits rarely pass without mentioning the disjunction between how the female medical student appears and what she actually feels. A favourite trope is

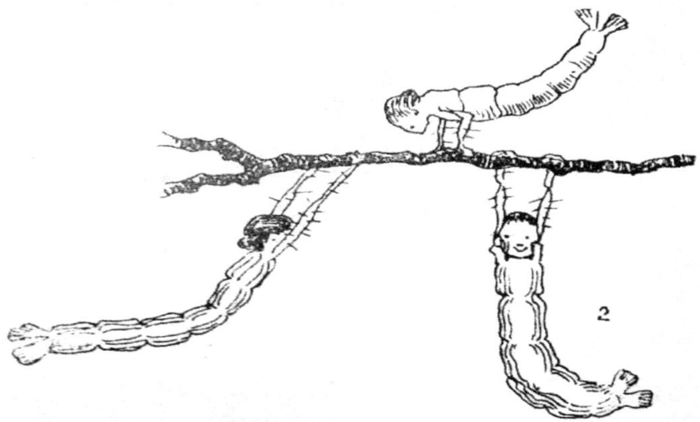

Aesculapia Athletica.

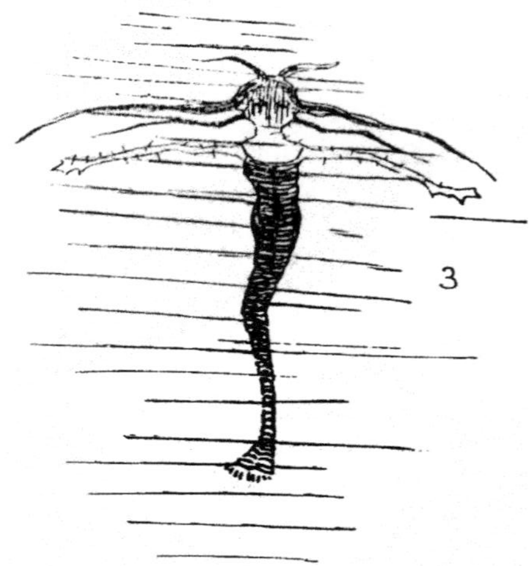

Aesculapia Aquatica.

Figure 8.2: 'Aesculapia Athletica' and 'Aesculapia Aquatica', in 'Some Notes on the Studentology of the Neighbourhood of Hunter Street and Gray's Inn Road (With Illustrations)', *LRFHSMWM*, 30 (January 1905), p. 427. Reproduced courtesy of the Royal Free Hospital Archive Centre, Royal Free London NHS Foundation Trust.

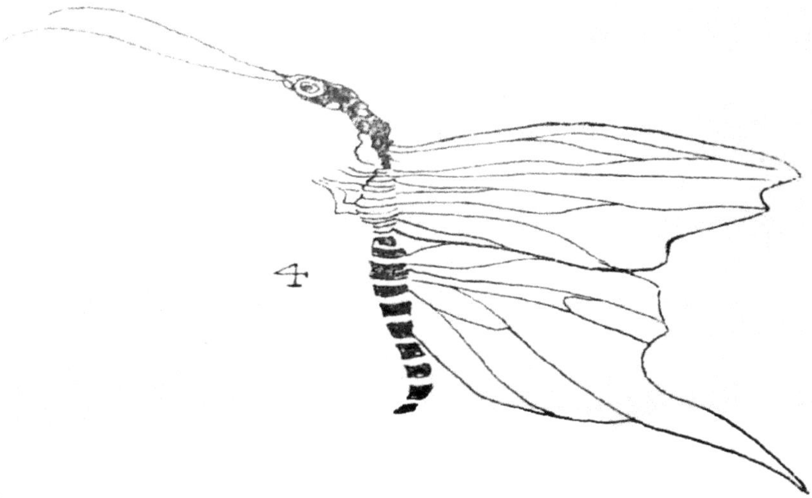

Figure 8.3: 'Vainessa Itinera', in 'Some Notes on the Studentology of the Neighbourhood of Hunter Street and Gray's Inn Road (With Illustrations)', p. 428. Reproduced courtesy of the Royal Free Hospital Archive Centre, Royal Free London NHS Foundation Trust. Text in 'Vainessa Itinera' image as in the original.

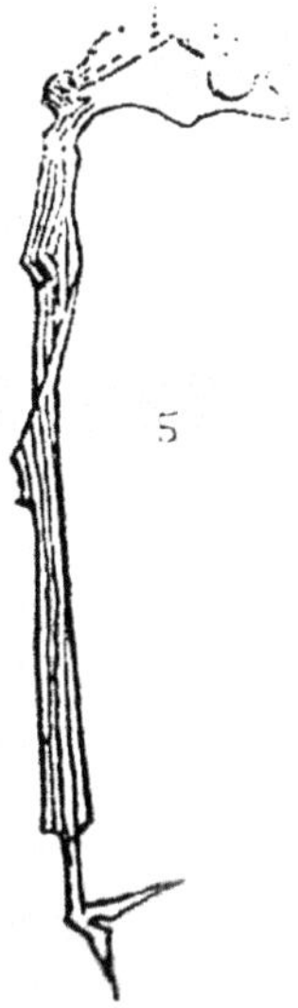

Figure 8.4: 'Antifeminina Inormata', in 'Some Notes on the Studentology of the Neighbourhood of Hunter Street and Gray's Inn Road (With Illustrations)', p. 428. Reproduced courtesy of the Royal Free Hospital Archive Centre, Royal Free London NHS Foundation Trust. Text in 'Antifeminina Inormata' image as in the original.

the use of decorations to disguise the reality of a medical school. To note just one example, a 1907 description of the annual School Party begins:

> The festive appearance of the various rooms bore witness to earlier activities, and such things as would offend the eye of the uninitiated were screened from view by draperies of varying hue and texture arranged in artistic folds. In the gay bower to which dancers led their fair partners who, but those who knew, could recognise the Museum – that habitation of dry bones? In the supper-room reserved for dancers, who would have suspected that behind choice hangings and decorations of ivy and flowers lurked deadly poisons in their stoppered bottles, flanked by material for producing the obnoxious odours which have gained for the science of chemistry the opprobrium of the multitude?[48]

Only the initiated are aware that just beneath the slight coverings lurk the horrors of the medical trade. The 'secret satisfaction' revealed here expresses both the female medical student's difference and unites her against others with her fellows.[49] Further humour is elicited at the expense of the outside world when accounts of parties, speeches or charity fundraising are accompanied by descriptions of the hosts' surprisingly ladylike appearances and skills. The Christmas Ward Entertainment at the Royal Free in 1906 had witnessed a variation on Gilbert and Sullivan's 'Three Little Maids', whereby six maids and another two 'Pretty Maids' had provided the entertainment. Strikingly, the latter was a 'characteristic anything but distinctive in such a gathering'.[50] Party preparations in a 1902 edition of the *Magazine* were prefaced with the following comment: 'Orthodox maiden aunts, and dowagers of both sexes (!) would have wept for joy to see the domestic knowledge displayed by apparently hardened and unregenerate medical students'.[51] Throughout the LSMW *Magazine*, female medical students revel in confounding the expectations of supporters and detractors alike. Pride can be garnered both from their medical achievements and their femininity. One need not preclude the other.

Indeed, it is the combination of the two which so delights the students themselves. On the surface, the female medical student is, in fact, indistinguishable from any other young woman, but look more closely and the marks of her trade will be evident. Branded by the profession: 'our zeal is evidenced by the crimson and orange stains with which we adorn our fingers, and the red-edged rents which splashes of sulphuric acid make in our gowns'.[52] This sense of camaraderie is perpetuated through the *Magazine* itself, which is literally part of the student body: an 'Organ of Special Sense', according to Miss Cock, who succeeded Elizabeth Garrett Anderson as the Dean of the LSMW.[53] A 'mirror of all that happened at School and at Hospital', the *Magazine* allowed past students to keep 'in touch with the present life', showing 'not only how the work is carried on, and how the scientific spirit is fostered, but also how outside interests have widened with the increase in the number of students'.[54] Indeed, the number of clubs and societies upon which the magazine reports, from professionally-based organizations such as the Medical Society, or the intra- and inter-collegiate battles between, among many others, hockey, swimming, fencing, rowing and debating clubs, reveals the female medical students' ability to band together formally and compete as a School. But this focus on 'outside' concerns, rather than bringing the student body – past and present – together also has the opposite effect and threatens to expose divisions in attitudes.

When discussing the purpose of the magazine, the older generation wished, nostalgically, 'to have the atmosphere of School and Hospital infused into the magazine' so that they could 'hear what the students were discussing among themselves, what, in short, was "the latest craze"'. This was so 'that they might feel, when they returned to their old haunts, that they were not altogether strangers in the land'.[55] Over the fifteen years covered by this essay, there are repeated calls for unity amongst medical women, suggesting that the bond between them was not as it should be. An annual dinner was established after a 1902 letter from former student, Eleanor C. Bond, who lamented the scant connection between the School and its alumni: 'I feel strongly', she urged, 'that such a gathering would tend to promote the sentiment of esprit de corps in which, perhaps, it is the failing of our sex to be a little wanting'.[56] Although numbers at the dinner reached 300 in 1903, by 1909 they were down to 158.[57] The 'pessimists' who prophesied that interest would wane were evidently not far wrong. That 'there will always be a certain number who will look forward to and count on the Annual Dinner as a fixed enjoyment' implied that there were others who would not.[58]

If the female medical body was fit enough to practise, esprit de corps, on the other hand, was wavering by 1910. Nowhere is this more evident than in the debate over co-education. The possibility of women being educated alongside men, companionably dissecting the human body together, horrified detractors, who feared the immorality which could result from such propinquity between the sexes. But by 1910, many of the older generation of medical women, and, indeed, some of the younger, were also arguing for the benefits of single-sex education, anxious to see the female medical student retain her identity and, consequently, her separate and unique status. A rumour about the London Hospital, from their own *Gazette*, concerning the possible admission of women students receives short shrift from the editor of the LSMW *Magazine*, M. A. Blair.[59] Speaking for the School, where there is 'no general demand' for such a move, Blair objects because she 'fail[s] to see that any further widening of the student experience is either necessary or desirable': 'we consider it more desirable that women should be trained apart from men'. Indeed, such a scheme could cause 'damage' to 'our own School of Medicine, where we consider that a woman may be most efficiently and most satisfactorily trained to fit herself for the work of a medical practitioner'.[60] The next issue of the *Magazine*, however, revealed that the editor was by no means voicing the only opinion. Support for her stance was evident in the annual opening address, this year given by the Royal Free surgeon, E. W. Roughton, who radically claimed, when arguing for the continued separation of the sexes, that even teaching staff should be exclusively female.[61] The address is unusually reproduced in full, a rare occurrence in the *Magazine* unless the topic is particularly pertinent or the speaker important. In the correspondence section, Gwendolyn M. Burns, keen to stress that the letter is '[her] opinion only', concurs with the opposition to any changes. It should be 'fully and fitly recognised', she notes, that 'our School' is 'unique': 'the record of those who have gone out before and have made our way easy for us seems to bear this out'. Two other correspondents, however, dispute the lack of demand for co-education. M. Forrester Brown, a 'junior Hospital student', reminds the older editor that her opinion, based on 'long experience' does 'not completely coincide with that of the majority of my contemporaries and of the more recent generations of students'. In fact, Forrester Brown and her friends 'look forward to co-education in all medical schools as an inevitable and desirable goal, and we heartily welcome each step in that direction'. Similarly, Olive Gray, the School sub-editor, suggests that '[a]ny enlargement of opportunities of medical study for women is desirable'.[62] The most 'fitting' route for medical women to practise was no longer an exclusive one. It had once been the only possibility, but now many had begun to feel stifled by the narrowness of the path.

By the end of the Edwardian period, cracks were appearing in the carefully moulded outline of the ideal female medical student. As the co-education debate showed, while some wanted to immerse themselves in the 'spirit' and 'atmosphere' of the School, others wanted room to breathe outside its walls. Women had proved they were more than capable of medical study and the moral, mental and physical demands of medical practice, but divisions were developing in the student body over the most 'fitting' route to successful careers. In the October 1910 edition of the LSMW *Magazine*, the poem 'No, thanks very much' condemned the tardy invitations to co-education with a defence of the all-female citadel:

> This should have come, you know,
> Many, many years ago,
> But to-day we need your generous help no more!
> ...
> So we send,
> As a friend,
> Many thanks. But to the end
> We prefer our Royal teaching and the rest.
> You may have a 1000 beds,
> But *we* reckon things by heads,
> And we're really quite contented with the best.[63]

Although the first generation of medical women had stormed the hills 'fortified by men', they had erected their own barriers at the LSMW and forged an image of an ideal. In a stronger position than ever before, by the 1910s, some female medical students were no longer strengthened by the insistence on standing alone. The outside was looking very welcoming to those invigorated by new possibilities of escaping the sheltering wing of the LSMW and exercising their prowess elsewhere.

9 UNSTABLE ADOLESCENCE/UNSTABLE LITERATURE? MANAGING BRITISH GIRLS' HEALTH AROUND 1900

Hilary Marland

As the nineteenth century came to an end, writer, physician and 'eugenic feminist', Dr Arabella Kenealy, regaled the readers of the literary magazine *Nineteenth Century* with the transformative story of Clara. A year ago, Clara could not walk more than two miles without tiring: 'now she can play tennis or hockey, or can bicycle all day without feeling it'. Through exercise and a vigorous lifestyle, Clara had toned and honed muscles, was slimmer, stronger and more agile. However, she had bartered many qualities for a 'mess of muscle' and lost her subtle charms in the process – sympathy, patience and elusive beauty. In their place Clara had developed a highly toned body, briskness, 'mere muscular achievement' and a 'bicycle face' (the face of muscular tension). She had a booming voice, neglected her domestic tasks and had abandoned 'gliding' in favour of 'manly striding'.[1] Clara had thus in Kenealy's view traded her femininity for a strident masculinity as she achieved robust health.

In contrast, just three years prior to Kenealy's pronouncements on Clara, the eminent London obstetrician and gynaecologist, Dr William Playfair, had praised English girls for setting good examples of health, citing 'Lawn Tennis Girl',

> an excellent example of the healthy, well-developed, and unsentimental girl – the girl who does not think it necessary to devote herself to the study of her own emotions, and who finds in active physical exercise an antidote to the morbid fancies which are too apt to creep into the mind of the idle and self-indulgent.[2]

His comments were made in a leading gynaecological textbook, but the descriptor 'Lawn Tennis Girl' and his quotation were lifted directly from an article describing the girl of today in an 1895 issue of *Speaker* magazine. 'Lawn Tennis Girl', unlike 'bicycle face Clara', had traded drooping femininity for a much-improved modern, energetic model of girlhood.

These two examples are significant – and to a certain extent confound our expectations about who was likely to say what about the ways in which the health of young women was pictured during the late Victorian period. The story of Clara was related by a female physician, an ardent and outspoken eugenicist; while claiming feminist credentials, Kenealy's concerns about relations between the sexes were prompted predominantly 'by anxiety about the future of the British race'.[3] In favour of moderate exercise for girls, she cautioned against over-exertion in athletics. Writing a preface to fellow eugenicist Dr Emma Walker's advice manual, *Beauty through Hygiene*, Kenealy warned girls about the risks of expending 'too large a share of our nervous force in athletic exercise', nerve force which was required for future investment in motherhood.[4] Kenealy's piece in *Nineteenth Century* insisted that Clara and her sister athletes were squandering 'the birthright of the babies', 'debasing her womanhood, in becoming a neuter', 'her children are nursed, fed, clothed, taught and trained by hirelings'.[5] Her article attracted considerable comment – not surprisingly, for Kenealy was considered outspoken and controversial by many, her views out of kilter with those of feminists, social reformers, educationalists and female doctors alike. The writer and feminist, Laura Ormiston Chant, responded in *Nineteenth Century* that female athleticism – rather than threatening the potential of the race – would lead to its improvement and embellishment.[6] An editorial in *Review of Reviews*, meanwhile, while suggesting that Keanely said much that was 'extremely sensible', claimed 'the net effect of her pleadings will be to encourage the belief that to be good mothers women must neither be well educated nor physically well trained'. It continued,

> Over-training, no doubt, in man or woman is bad. But not being trained at all is worse. The women of to-day are undoubtedly by universal consent finer physically, healthier, taller, more vigorous than were Miss Lydia Languish and her sisters of last century. And it is impossible to believe that this improved physique does not react favourably upon My Lord the Baby.[7]

After twenty-five years as Professor of Obstetric Medicine at King's College and obstetric physician to King's College Hospital, Playfair was also preoccupied with women's preparedness for motherhood.[8] Elsewhere – as will be demonstrated later – he expressed concern about the impact of study on young women's health, and he thus put out mixed messages on women's potential to thrive, or alternatively, to face physical and mental breakdown when confronted with the challenges of new opportunities at school or on the sports field. Playfair had imported Dr Silas Weir Mitchell's rest cure for neurasthenia into Britain in the 1880s, and a good portion of his lucrative private practice focused on his treatment of cases of nervous exhaustion or neurasthenia, which claimed as its victims many young women in transition from domestic to professional roles. Yet here, writing in a mainstream gynaecological textbook, he firmly advocated girls' outdoor pursuits as enabling and improving. Playfair's choice of tennis as a sport that would bolster the health and well-being of girls was an interesting one and supported by other medical commentators who placed tennis high up in the hierarchy of appropriate sports for young women. As one contributor to the *Practitioner* exclaimed in 1895, 'it would be deplorable if girls whom lawn-tennis has made, like daughters of the gods, divinely tall should be made humpbacked by the bicycle!'[9]

These two examples illuminate the complex relationships between medical and lay publications and medical and lay audiences, and the fluidity of the passage of ideas, arguments and depictions of girls' health between medical and lay spheres. While Kenealy bemoaned the fact that 'public opinion sets its face against the discussing of physiological questions in any but medical journals', her article in fact generated a robust response in *Nineteenth Century* and in other magazines and journals in the weeks that followed its publication.[10] This leaching of medical writing into public media was commonplace rather than exceptional during this period, and many medical authors published in both mainstream medical journals and general interest or literary publications.[11] Meanwhile, Playfair's textbook commentary on 'Lawn Tennis Girl' was intended predominantly, one imagines, for medical colleagues and students, but the phraseology and general thrust of his piece was closely based on what he had read in an editorial intended for a lay readership.

This chapter explores the ways in which debates on the health of young women were reflected in a diverse set of publications in equally diverse ways around 1900. It also underlines how interconnected medicine was with concerns about the new avenues in education, work, public life, leisure and sporting activities that were opening up to girls in this period. While Anne Digby and others have emphasized the ways in which biological determinism gained particular resonance by the mid-nineteenth century, spurred on by the new specialist fields of gynaecology and psychiatry, the period around 1900 was perhaps even more notable not only for the direct engagement of physicians with the fortunes of young women but for the rapid proliferation of a literature on this subject in a multiplicity of print outlets.[12]

The Perils of Puberty

The late Victorian era was ostensibly one typified by rigid and doom-ridden medical opinion on the subject of women's and girls' health, imbued with theories of degeneration and biological determinism, topped up towards the end of the century by eugenicist concerns and anxieties about the future of the race and nation, and laced with worries about the ambitions of young women to engage in new social, educational and political endeavours. It is easy enough to locate grim pronouncements, chilling accounts of the dangers waiting for every high school girl, cyclist, New Woman or would-be suffragist – weakness and sickness, diseased and decaying body parts, neuroses and mental illness, loss of charm and character and an inability – physically and emotionally – to take on the duties of motherhood. Women were liable to be configured in medical discourse throughout the Victorian and Edwardian periods as disordered and deviant in behaviour as well as bodily and mental state, and girls particularly so, having the added instability of female adolescence to contend with. Many doctors were minded to prescribe limits to girls' activities given the health risks they imposed at such a vulnerable time, and in particular warned that the expenditure of vitality was likely to imperil future motherhood.

Hysteria, 'the daughter's disease', was discussed and debated with great frequency in medical and lay literature during the latter decades of the nineteenth century, accompanied by specific case histories. Anorexia nervosa too gained considerable attention, as exemplified by Susannah Wilson in this collection. Both hysteria and anorexia were reputed to envelop girls in a cycle of disruptive behaviour, violation of the laws of health, and physiological and nervous collapse. Playfair attributed many cases of anorexia to overstrain and 'severe study' as well as over-athletic activity.[13] In 1880 Dr J. Mortimer-Granville, best known as the inventor of the electric vibrator, and an authority and well-cited author on lunacy and its management, warned parents and guardians in no uncertain terms about the dangers of the 'girl-youth'.[14] Mortimer-Granville cautioned parents to watch for indications of illness, disease or special weakness, especially if there was a hereditary taint in the family. Girls, he claimed, were prone to palpitations, hysterics, fainting fits, giddiness, blood disorders, outbursts of temper, moodiness, nocturnal tooth grinding, nightmares and sleepwalking. A hysterical cough likely signalled consumption, growing pains indicated incipient rheumatism, and stooping was a sign of deformity of the spine and limbs.[15] Mortimer-Granville's 'awkward age' could be short or prolonged, and be marked by a 'vague expression of weariness and ungainly stupidity or sullenness'; 'a courteous demeanour may conceal an ungracious heart: an attractive and innocent surface-character made up of smiles and pleasing manners, may veil a repellent and vicious nature'.[16] Boys too were liable to suffer during puberty, were corruptible and likely to go astray, lazy, untruthful, moody, 'girlish' or weakly. But girls faced the additional challenge of menstruation at puberty, and were described as excessively vulnerable and rather sinister.

Other medical authors added further warnings on how the mismanagement of adolescence – and particularly the onset of menstruation – was likely to have dire consequences for young women. Dr George Black's *Young Wife's Advice Book* explained how 'a lazy, listless life; undue mental excitement, either caused by the reading of sensational novels, by conversation or the like; late hours, irregular habits of sleep, highly seasoned articles of diet, and stimulants, have all a tendency to accelerate the occurrence of menstruation', something many medical authors wished to avoid at all costs.[17] In 1851 Dr Edward Tilt had urged the retardation of menstruation and believed that its monthly reoccurrence weighed heavily on girls' spirits and gave rise to nervousness and hysteria.[18] In 1882 Dr Lionel Weatherly cautioned in his *The Young Wife's Own Book* against following music lessons during menstruation, as sitting upright with the back unsupported and 'drumming vigorously' on the piano was detrimental and resulted in 'strong excitement of the emotions'.[19] Poorly managed menstruation was a frequent cause of hysteria and other disorders, and drew evocative descriptions from authors such as Weatherly:

> The number of colourless, pale-complexioned, short-breathed, and sickly-looking girls that are ever to be seen, own their condition, in nineteen cases out of twenty, to some unhealthy form of menstruation, which if not taken in time may soon land the poor creatures into a consumption.[20]

Eugenicist physician Robert Reid Rentoul described puberty as a time of unprecedented risk for girls; they were fragile beings and the passage into womanhood a time of grave danger;

> a girl when becoming a woman should not have any mental or bodily labour to perform. She should therefore neither study nor work, but have only good food, exercise, sleep, and clothing. If she accomplishes the beginning of this important phase of her life with vigour and success, she will have secured one of the chief ends of her existence.[21]

'The effort to develop into womanhood requires all the best energies and strength a girl can possess', Rentoul concluded.[22] Dire consequences were likely to follow if these recommendations were not obeyed: weakness, disability and even death.

The Diversity of Health Literature

If we delve deeper into the medical literature and that produced for a wider readership on health matters (which, as we have noted, might have fairly fluid boundaries, in terms of the passage of information to and fro) – read it more carefully and at first hand – a more complicated set of attitudes towards the health status of women and adolescent girls emerges. This was paralleled by an array of advice, admonition and instruction on how to preserve and improve health, much of which directly addressed the ways in which young women could maximize their potential to engage in new activities. Medical texts and health advice literature reveal subtle and complex approaches to dealing with girls' health. A number of doctors – including those who have been singled out as presenting a particularly gloomy and misogynistic viewpoint – were willing to explore the potential for girls to improve their health status, albeit moderately and incrementally, with a view to protecting their health for future marriage and motherhood.

The late nineteenth century was marked by intense engagement on the part of medical men with lay audiences and the opening up of new channels of communication. There was nothing new, of course, in doctors writing for a variety of potential readers, for example, in household medical guides and guides to new mothers – and in so doing bolstering their medical income and reputation – but the production of prescriptive literature stepped up considerably towards the end of the century, as did the expansion of outlets for expressing medical viewpoints.[23] The nineteenth century was the 'age of Periodicals' – and many focused on health in their features articles and advice columns. As Karen Flint has argued,

> hypothesis about the assumed connections between psychology and physiology passed readily from specialist scientific research into more widely circulating discourse ... aided by the publication of many of the medical findings not in specialist journals, but in magazines with a far broader readership.[24]

And within these magazines, young women's health featured particularly strongly, as magazines catering directly for this audience also proliferated, supplementing those targeting wider female readership groups and relating health issues to the new range of challenges and activities opening up to girls.[25]

With regard to some media it is difficult to distinguish one from the other in terms of labelling them 'medical' or 'lay'. Medical periodicals and textbooks are easy to categorize as 'medical', while women's and girls' magazines, for example, are clearly 'lay'. But moving in between these was a large amount of prescriptive literature in the form of articles, pamphlets and advice manuals, produced not only by doctors – including an increasing number of women doctors – but also journalists, headmistresses and teachers, activists in voluntary associations and clubs, welfare supervisors, and sportsmen and women. Numerous articles in the periodical press and newspapers, women's and girls' magazines, and girls' annuals offered advice as well as space for medical debates and letters from readers. Health guides for girls were part of a much broader expansion, meanwhile, of a literature for girls, much speaking directly to them rather than via their mothers.[26] Health manuals ranged from slim illustrated volumes offering chatty tips on beauty, deportment and exercise to dense, stolid tomes barely distinguishable from medical textbooks covering physiology, nutrition, hygiene and public health, sick nursing and child care, such as Elizabeth Sloan Chesser's *Physiology and Hygiene for Girls' Schools and Colleges*, a 'comprehensive training' for girls to 'fit them to be efficient in the home sphere',[27] and Malcolm Morris's bulky *The Book of Health*, intended 'to place before the general reader, in an intelligible form ... the principal rules that should be adopted for the preservation of Health'.[28] Thus there was a rapidly expanding, diversifying and complex range of outlets for medical views and medical advice, which enabled doctors to line their pockets and broaden their public profiles, giving to them enormous potential to influence as well as inform.

Doctors increasingly opted to publish keynote articles in lay periodicals, in a conscious decision, one imagines, to relay their knowledge and viewpoints to as wide an audience as possible, in an era when advertising by doctors was increasingly restricted by their professional associations and codes of practice. Kenealy chose to publish her views on the female athlete, cited above, in *Nineteenth Century* rather than a medical journal, while some twenty years previously, in 1874, eminent British psychiatrist Henry Maudsley had published his controversial and highly influential article, 'Sex in Mind and in Education' in the *Fortnightly Review*, rather than the *Lancet*, *British Medical Journal* or the *Journal of Mental Science*, which he himself edited.[29] Maudsley's article triggered an immediate and energetic response from Dr Elizabeth Garrett Anderson, the first women to qualify as a physician and surgeon in Britain, published in the subsequent issue of the *Fortnightly Review*, and the debate on young women's competence to enter higher education, which was at the core of this exchange, would continue to reverberate through the medical and lay press for decades to come.[30] Medical journalism would comprise a major aspect of the work of many physicians, including growing numbers of women doctors. Dr Elizabeth Sloan Chesser exemplified this trend; her numerous publications on motherhood and the health and vitality of women, to be briefly explored in the final section of this chapter, appeared in the form of health guides and articles in popular magazines and newspapers.

Unstable Literatures

This incursion of medical authorship into lay outlets could be interpreted as the extension and application of medical theories to ways of life and public and private arenas and activities that had previously been largely independent of this form of intervention. Such literature certainly spoke to debates about the participation of women and girls in public life, education, work and sport, and leisure. But it did more than this, and, in effect, much turned on and challenged dominant medical theories and practices which represented girls as physically and mentally weak and incapable.

One theory in particular dominated views on women's capacity for health in the late nineteenth century, which was given enormous impetus by Henry Maudsley's article, 'Sex in Mind and in Education': that young women could call on only limited supplies of energy to fuel their physical and mental activities. By the third quarter of the nineteenth century medical practitioners, notably gynaecologists and psychiatrists, had evolved an 'economic' model to explain how women's reproductive systems interacted with other parts of the body, especially the brain, depicting

> the body as a closed system in which organs and mental faculties competed for a finite supply of physical or mental energy; thus stimulation or depletion in one organ resulted in exhaustion or excitation in another part of the body.[31]

The two high priests of the 'fixed fund of energy' theory, Harvard Professor Edward H. Clarke and Maudsley, were remarkably successful in propagating their ideas on both sides of the Atlantic. According to Clarke, excessive physical or mental labour would reduce the supply of nerve energy to the female reproductive system, and put schoolgirls at risk of injury to health, neuralgia, uterine disease, hysteria and other derangements of the nervous system.[32] If education interfered with the establishment of healthy, regular menstruation, according to Clarke, it could result in halted development, with girls graduating 'from school or college excellent scholars, but with underdeveloped ovaries'.[33] Maudsley explained in the *Fortnightly Review* how overspending vital energy threatened to cause menstrual disorders and mental breakdown, and potentially would destroy women's capacity to bear healthy children. Women should not attempt to run alongside men, Maudsley famously declared: 'They cannot choose but to be women; cannot rebel successfully against the tyranny of their organization'. 'The important physiological change which takes place at puberty ... may easily overstep its health limits, and pass into pathological change.'[34] Elsewhere, however, Maudsley – rather surprisingly – framed female adolescence as rather more complicated. He suggested that girls suffered more than boys during this epoch, not just because of the influence of their reproductive organs and the challenge of menstruation, but also because 'the range of activity of women is so limited, and their available paths of work in life so few ... they have not like men, vicarious outlets for feeling in a variety of aims and health pursuits'.[35] Thus while Maudsley drew on biology to support his often pessimistic diatribes on girls' capacity for ill health, he was prepared to acknowledge that ill health could potentially result from underactivity and boredom.

Hysteria in adolescent girls of the 'comfortable classes' was a source of rich copy in medical and popular literature.[36] Psychiatrist F. C. Skey argued that hysteria was 'most prevalent in the young female members of the higher and middle classes, of such as live a life of ease and luxury, those who have limited responsibilities in life, of no compelled occupation, and who have both time and inclination to indulge in the world's pleasures – persons easily excited to mental emotion, of sensitive feeling, often delicate and refined'.[37] Such women were not necessarily weak minded, Skey added: 'It will often select for its victim a female member of a family exhibiting more than usual force and decision of character, of strong resolution, fearless of danger, bold riders, having plenty of what is termed *nerve*'.[38] Dr Horatio Bryan Donkin, neurologist, progressive thinker, and doctor to Karl Marx and the feminist author Olive Schreiner, provided a complex reading of hysteria in his 1892 essay, outlining the social and sexual restrictions that made young women liable to mental disorders. He agreed that hysteria was most likely to afflict young women, subject to nervous imbalance triggered by enormous physical changes particularly in her sexual organs, but her social condition and the frustrations this entailed were also of great relevance:

> The nervous balance is thus in especially unstable equilibrium. With this greater internal stress on the nervous organism there are in the surroundings and general training of most girls many hindrances to the retention or restoration of due stability and but few channels of outlet for her new activities. It is not only in the educational repression and ignorance as regards sexual matters of which she is the subject that this difference is manifest, but all kinds of other barriers to the free play of her powers are set up by ordinary social and ethical customs. 'Thou shall not' meets a girl at almost every turn. The exceptions to this rule are found in those instances of good education or necessity, or both, have regular work and definite pursuits.[39]

This compared with conditions for the young man, 'whose comparative freedom and the various and necessary occupations ... offer many safety valves for his comparatively minor nervous tension'.[40] The ferocity and impact of hysteria tended to be dampened down in prescriptive literature and lay periodicals, where it was also described and analysed avidly. Dr A. T. Schofield, a regular contributor on a variety of topics pertaining to girl's health, described in *Leisure Hour* how hysteria's victims were typically under-worked, unhappy, suffering mental strain, exposed to excessive luxury or an ill-balanced education. The cure was straightforward: to feel 'true sympathy from the conviction of the reality of the disease, but showing none'.[41] Schofield's description of hysteria closely mirrored that of Skey, emphasizing that the condition manifested itself in those with strong minds with plenty of nerve. For medical author and editor Dr Andrew Wilson, writing in the popular periodical *Health*, 'a glass of cold water suddenly dashed in the patient's face' helped, as did 'fresh air, exercise and health pursuits to engage body and mind'.[42]

A careful reading of medical texts indicates the existence of other more balanced and considered views on women's and girls' health issues, and pragmatic suggestions on health improvement. Even Dr Edward Tilt, who has emerged as something of a bête noire of Victorian womanhood, included constructive, practical advice alongside his warnings about the dangers of menstruation and the associated risks of operas, novels and lounging on sofas. He insisted that mothers should never let a girl be taken unawares at the onset of puberty, or put girls on shortened allowances of food or limit outdoor exercise to them, which he referred to as 'bedlamite conduct'. Tilt encouraged a rounded education for girls and criticized poor levels of attention to health and exercise at girls' schools.[43] One of the most prolific authors of domestic health guides and advice literature, Dr J. H. Walsh, suggested that, while it could be affected by poor health, menstruation itself was normally a healthy process. He urged mothers to inform their daughters about the changes wrought by puberty; otherwise their daughters might not only feel shame about menstruation but also attempt to repress it.[44] The durable advice offered by Henry Chavasse to women and girls, which passed through numerous editions in the late nineteenth and early twentieth centuries, insisted that the onset of menstruation should be taken as a natural occurrence, unmarked by pain, sickness or invalidism. Chavasse urged attention to 'Nature's laws', and cited the principle causes of weakness, nerves and unhappiness as 'ignorance of the laws of health, Nature's laws being set at nought by fashion and by folly, by want of fresh air and exercise, by want of occupation, and by want of self-reliance'.[45] He approved a range of exercises, including horse riding, the 'glorious game' of croquet and archery.[46]

We have already heard Playfair's views on 'Lawn Tennis Girl', which contrasted strikingly with his negative comments on young female anorexics and hysterics, described as 'thoroughly enjoying their life of inert self-indulgence'.[47] Hysterics, however, were themselves compared with neurasthenics who were lauded for their femininity and delicacy, and their efforts to get better, unlike the grasping, selfish hysteric. Addressing the fixed fund of energy theory and the question of the relationship between over-study and female health, Playfair complained of cases of schools with little or no provision for exercise, that ignored their duty of care in inquiring into the health of their pupils and urged their pupils to work at their studies for seven to eight hours a day. Playfair suggested that moderate exercise and attention to health combined with fewer hours of study was entirely appropriate and would, in most cases, serve to preserve young women's health.[48] He warned against girls being raised 'like hothouse plants' which would leave a 'wretched broken-down invalid', and urged headmistresses to engage with medical advice rather than accusing medical men of 'narrow-mindedness and opposition'.[49] Parents and teachers were reminded in 1905 by Dr Clement Dukes, physician to Rugby School, in an essay on the hygiene of youth to 'instil into girls' minds that fact that it is their duty to be physically strong, and to provide for its attainment by adequate means', principally exercise. Dukes argued that a more 'reasonable system' of training would banish nerves and fainting in girls.[50] In this he echoed the opinions of headmistresses and feminists, eager to promote higher education for girls and to present ways in which it could be conducted to enhance rather than imperil health.

Meanwhile, girls' magazines increasingly conveyed positive health messages. The *Girl's Own Paper* (*GOP*), though publishing often contradictory pieces on the questions of girls' status, prospects, careers and ideal demeanour, produced a regular advice column, edited for thirty years by Dr Gordon Stables, ex-naval surgeon, prolific author of prescriptive health literature and adventure stories for boys, and writer of a similar column in the *Boy's Own Paper*. Stables's advice was of the straightforward, no-nonsense variety: cold baths, hot porridge, brisk exercise and early to bed. He busied himself with preparing his girl readers for an active life, involving charity work, sick nursing, games and physical activity. He acknowledged that poorer girls were often compelled to work, though was cagey about whether other girls should do likewise. He concluded that the majority of the readership of *GOP* was 'healthy in lungs and nerves, and ... stout-hearted and strong-limbed'.[51] Stables's girls were encouraged to be fit and strong; 'the muscles should be hard and firm, maintained by gymnasium work and callisthenics'.[52] He likened suggestions that girls need not exercise and should stand by and watch 'their brothers or friends show off their prowess on the field, or in the gymnasium' to fairy stories. 'But those days have gone by, never to return, because we know now that there can be neither health nor perfect happiness in a feeble or badly developed body or frame'.[53] Good character went hand in hand with good health, according to Stables, who demanded a certain amount of pluckiness from his readers as well as a regard for correct principles as these applied to behaviour and rules of health; he instructed his readers to 'Keep a smiling face .... fretting weakens the body',[54] and stated that 'The mind has much to do with the health of the body. Try to control your temper, never get angry ... Read good books, especially religious books'.[55]

Gordon Stables ascribed to a straightforward theory on energy supply, at odds with the 'fixed fund of energy' thesis and the pronouncements of many of his professional colleagues. He advised in 1885 that some girls had the potential for more improvement than others, with 'depressive and nervous girls', that is, middle-class girls with no employment outside the home, being cautioned to be careful in their approach to exercise.[56] Working girls were depicted as being more robust, their energy a form of capital to be built upon. Yet they were also warned – despite the economic imperative to work – not to over-exert themselves and to take proper nourishment, rest and outdoor exercise, something, Stables failed to recognize, that many such girls were not at liberty to do.[57] Stables acknowledged the scope for incremental improvement for all young women: 'All kinds of exercise do good; walking for the weakly, cycling and rowing for the stronger, the dumb-bells and Indian clubs before breakfast or in the afternoon for all'.[58] Yet for Stables – and many other medical authors – the turn of the century was marked by new anxieties about the relationship between girls' health, exercise and motherhood; girls were becoming too ambitious and rejecting their futures as mothers of the Empire. In 1901 he urged readers of the *GOP* 'not to have too much of that Emancipation business'. 'Who wants a girl with biceps, anyhow? ... Your women who scull much, or golf or hockey a deal are usually coarse in skin and in features, and far indeed from beautiful.'[59] In contrast with earlier pronouncements advocating that girls shared in the sporting activities of their brothers, Stables denounced 'man-games and tom-boy exercises' that would result in their loss of womanly elegance.[60]

The modern girl, lauded for substituting the wan, weakly and nervous Victorian girl-type, was at risk of being replaced by a new danger. The *Speaker* warned that while 'Lawn Tennis Girl' had 'driven out the old-fashioned style of heroine – the slim maiden who was ready to faint' she has herself been beaten for a time by the 'unwholesome travesty of her sex who now usurps the title of "the new woman"'.[61] While Arabella Kenealy's views were seen by some as extreme and wrong-headed, she did keep the attention of many medical commentators in spelling out the risks of overexertion and the too-active pursuit of education and physical excellence, and, unlike many other medical authors, she did not waver in her views. Yet, by the cusp of the First World War, when national concerns and anxieties about the future of the race were at their height, other medical authors were asserting that women had the ability to harness and husband energy effectively, and girls were described as able to flourish as scholars and athletes and then still to become good mothers. Dr Florence Richards described in *Hygiene for Girls* in 1913 how

> The best exercise is that which combines some special object to be attained with the exercising of the muscles. The mind is thus stimulated, and consequently muscles and nerves work harmoniously together. Thus useful labour and games having some other object than mere exercise, neither over-tax the nerves nor exhaust the will power.[62]

In the same year Dr Elizabeth Sloan Chesser warned of the dangers of over-fatigue, but equally suggested:

> We have all got a reserve of energy that can be drawn upon, but it is never wise to *over*-draw our health account. We should rather, by studying health and hygiene, by good management of our hours of work and our hours of leisure, conserve our energies and expend them to our best advantage.[63]

Chesser was best known for her work as a medical journalist, building her reputation on the production of an array of books, articles in popular periodicals, women's magazines and newspapers, including the *National Review*, *Quiver*, *Good Housekeeping*, *Woman's Pictorial*, *Daily Express*, *Sunday Express* and *Glasgow Herald*.[64] Most of her books focused on women, their life cycles and health, and she was particularly interested in health and motherhood, seeing mothers and children as national assets, and was concerned to build a fit and efficient race. However, in sharp contrast to Kenealy, she was keen that girls – in the space between completing schooling and becoming wives and mothers – would occupy themselves creatively and usefully. While Kenealy applauded lassitude and rest during this period, Chesser decried idleness as morally, physically and mentally corrupting. As Greta Jones has suggested, Chesser's eugenicist credentials and emphasis on the importance of motherhood and domestic work did not come at the cost of women's exclusion from public and professional life and work outside the home.[65]

The 'secret of health', Chesser argued, 'is the wise expenditure of the energy of life forces we possess'.[66] For girls in transition – youth – this entailed, for example, the management of excessive expenditure of energy in games: 'No girl can afford to over-tire herself by games when she has important examinations in view'.[67] She disputed the ideas that girls who took up work outside the home lost their 'sweet "femininity"' and regretted women's lost lives in the 'old days' when they had no outlet for their energy and ability, their long years of 'vegetable existence'.[68] She claimed that the years from seventeen to twenty-two are the most valuable from an educational standpoint and must not be wasted:

> The girl whose days are filled with a few home duties which do not entail one hour of honest labour, with a little visiting and shopping, and a great deal of social recreation is not a healthy girl. She is stagnating mentally, morally. She is living a profitless existence, a stupid, aimless life which is essentially unhealthy.[69]

Chesser advocated a variety of useful occupations – including scientific training in housewifery – to fill these years, as well as 'preparing for University degrees, for some of the higher examinations, in training for the Civil Service or for gardening, art, music or some of the appointments available in the educational world'.[70] The balance between mental and physical activity, work and meaningful recreation, was one of the 'principles of health':

> *Mental exercise*, or intellectual work, is another factor in personal hygiene. A girl must do a certain amount of mental work if she is to keep in health. There are very real dangers in idleness. In the first place, a girl who has 'nothing to do' dissipates her energies in the futilities and trivialities of her life. If she has not got some real work on hand, she may spend her energy on undesirable occupations, or gradually come to find idleness supportable. This is the beginning of deterioration in character.[71]

Conclusion

Girls' health in the late Victorian and Edwardian periods was pictured by some medical authors as being on a knife edge as they traversed puberty, with many forms of disturbance liable to tip them into ill health, weakness, invalidism, insanity, sexual depravity and even death, or, yet worse, challenge their ability to develop as mothers, in terms of both physical and mental preparation. Yet by the turn of the century, preceding the physical culture movements of the 1920s and 1930s which have been presented as turning points in expectations about the bodies of young women, there was extensive debate – varied and invigorated – about the health of young women and its relationship to physical and mental activity, and in particular the use of energy as an asset for individual improvement and/or investment in future motherhood.[72] What we see if not the deadweight of medical theory imposing itself on women and girls, and restricting their activities, but rather lively discussion and an unstable set of views, unstable in the sense that doctors contradicted themselves on an apparently regular basis, as well as in the variety of opinions put forward, as the information traversed medical and public boundaries.

NOTES

Scott, Scarth and Chung, 'Introduction: Picturing Women's Health'

1. *OED*.
2. *OED*.
3. *OED*.
4. *OED*. Here we are using Wittgenstein's idea that pictures and language (proposition) represent states of affairs.
5. L. J. Jordanova, *Sexual Visions: Images of Gender in Science and Medicine between the Eighteenth and Twentieth Centuries* (Madison, WI: University of Wisconsin Press, 1989), p. 2.
6. J. M. Caldwell, *Literature and Medicine in Nineteenth-Century Britain: From Mary Shelley to George Eliot* (Cambridge: Cambridge University Press, 2004), p. 21.
7. J. Wiltshire, *Jane Austen and the Body: 'The Picture of Health'* (Cambridge: Cambridge University Press, 1992).
8. J. Austen, *Emma* (1815; London: Oxford University Press, 1966), p. 39.
9. Wiltshire, *Jane Austen and the Body*, p. 134.
10. Austen, *Emma*, p. 5.
11. J. Austen, *Mansfield Park*, in *The Complete Novels of Jane Austen* (1814; London: Penguin, 1996), p. 520.
12. M. Wollstonecraft, *A Vindication of the Rights of Woman*, in D. L. Macdondald and K. Scherf (eds), *The Vindications: The Rights of Men and the Rights of Woman* (1792; Ontario: Broadview Press, 2001), pp. 99–344, on p. 111.
13. Ibid., pp. 112, 195.
14. Ibid., p. 149.
15. Ibid., p. 306.
16. M. Brody, 'The Vindication of the Writes of Women: Mary Wollstonecraft and Enlightenment Rhetoric', in M. J. Falco (ed.), *Feminist Interpretations of Mary Wollstonecraft* (University Park, PA: Penn State Press, 2010), pp. 105–23, on p. 116.
17. A. Craciun, 'Violence against Difference: Mary Wollstonecraft and Mary Robinson', in G. Clingham (ed.), *Making History: Textuality and the Forms of Eighteenth Century Culture* (Cranbury and London: Associated University Presses, 1998), pp. 1–167, on p. 83.
18. Wollstonecraft, *Rights of Woman*, pp. 137, 163.
19. Ibid., p. 306.
20. Ibid.
21. Ibid., p. 315.

22. C. Macaulay, *Letters on Education: With Observations on Religious and Metaphysical Subjects* (London: C. Dilly, 1790), p. 136.
23. J. Sharp, *The Midwives Book, Or the Whole Art of Midwifery Discovered*, ed. E. Hobby (Oxford: Oxford University Press, 1999), p. 6.
24. Ibid.
25. Jordanova, *Sexual Visions*, p. 62.
26. T. Laqueur, *Making Sex: Body and Gender From the Greeks to Freud* (Cambridge, MA: Harvard University Press, 1990); K. Park and R. A. Nye, 'Destiny Is Anatomy', *New Republic* (18 February 1991), pp. 53–7.
27. J. Butler, *Personal Reminiscences of a Great Crusade* (London: Horace Marshall & Son, 1896), p. 18.
28. M. Kirkham (ed.), *Exploring the Dirty Side of Women's Health* (London and New York: Routledge, 2007), p. 236.
29. J. R. Walkowitz, *Prostitution and Victorian Society: Women, Class, and the State* (Cambridge: Cambridge University Press, 1982), p. 70.
30. L. Talairach-Velmas, *Moulding the Female Body in Victorian Fairy Tales and Sensation Novels* (Hampshire: Ashgate Publishing Ltd, 2007), p. 34.
31. D. Holbrook, *Charles Dickens and the Image of Women* (New York and London: New York University Press, 1993), p. 68.
32. S. Shuttleworth, *Charlotte Brontë and Victorian Psychology* (Cambridge: Cambridge University Press, 1996), p. 91.
33. See D. Flood, 'Blood and Transfusion in Bram Stoker's Dracula', *University of Mississippi Studies in English*, 7 (1989), pp. 180–92.
34. M. Jacobus, E. Fox Keller and S. Shuttleworth (eds), *Body/Politics: Women and the Discourses of Science* (New York and London: Routledge, 1990), p. 60.
35. See Matthew Arnold's 'On Literature and Science' (1882), written in response to Thomas Huxley's lecture 'Science and Culture' (1880). *The Complete Prose Works of Matthew Arnold*, ed. R. Super, 11 vols (Ann Arbor, MI: University of Michigan Press, 1974), vol. 10.
36. A. Mangham, '"What Could I Do?" Nineteenth-Century Psychology and the Horrors of Masculinity in *The Woman in White*', in K. Harrison and R. Fantina (eds), *Victorian Sensations: Essays on a Scandalous Genre* (Columbus, OH: Ohio State University Press, 2006), pp. 115–25, on p. 117.
37. Talairach-Velmas, *Moulding the Female Body*, p. 35.
38. M. H. Frawley, *Invalidism and Identity in Nineteenth-Century Britain* (Chicago, IL: University of Chicago Press, 2004), p. 49.
39. L. Duffin, 'The Conspicuous Consumptive', in L. Duffin and S. Delamont (eds), *The Nineteenth-Century Woman: Her Cultural and Physical World* (London: Routledge, 1978), pp. 26–56, on p. 26.
40. Ibid.
41. S. Roberts, *Sophia Jex-Blake: A Woman Pioneer in Nineteenth-Century Medical Reform* (London: Routledge, 2005), p. 2.
42. L. Appignanesi, *Mad, Bad and Sad: A History of Woman and the Mind Doctors from 1800* (London: Hachette Digital, 2008), p. 438.
43. See, for example, Shuttleworth, *Charlotte Brontë and Victorian Psychology*, M. W. Carpenter, *Imperial Bibles, Domestic Bodies: Women, Sexuality and Religion in the Victorian Market* (Athens, OH: Ohio University Press, 2003), H. Marland, *Dangerous Mother-*

hood: Insanity and Childbirth in Victorian Britain (New York: Palgrave Macmillan, 2004).

44. See, for example, M. W. Carpenter, 'Victorian Women as Patients and Practitioners', in M. W. Carpenter, *Health, Medicine and Society in Victorian England* (Connecticut: ABC-CLIO, 2010), pp. 149–75.
45. R. Cooter, 'The Traffic in Victorian Bodies: Medicine, Literature, and History', *Victorian Studies*, 45:3 (2003), pp. 513–27, on p. 514.
46. Ibid., p. 515.

1 Morrissey, 'Sensibility and Good Health in Charlotte Smith's *Ethelinde*'

1. G. J. Barker-Benfield, *The Culture of Sensibility: Sex and Society in Eighteenth-Century Britain* (Chicago, IL, and London: University of Chicago Press, 1992), p. 9.
2. Ibid., p. 28.
3. J. Spencer, 'Evelina and Cecilia', in *The Cambridge Companion to Francis Burney*, ed. P. Sabor (Cambridge: Cambridge University Press, 2007), pp. 23–37, on p. 35.
4. Ibid.
5. Ibid., p. 36.
6. C. Smith, *Ethelinde, or the Recluse of the Lake*, ed. S. Curran (1789; London: Pickering & Chatto, 2005), p. 208.
7. Ibid., p. 237.
8. See M. Butler, *Jane Austen and War of Ideas* (Oxford: Clarendon Press, 1975).
9. Smith, *Ethelinde*, p. 37.
10. Ibid.
11. Ibid.
12. Ibid.
13. Ibid.
14. Barker-Benfield, *The Culture of Sensibility*, p. 27.
15. Smith, *Ethelinde*, p. 45.
16. Ibid.
17. Ibid., p. 36.
18. Ibid., p. 28.
19. Ibid., p. 77.
20. Ibid.
21. Ibid., p. 351.
22. Ibid., p. 77.
23. Ibid., p. 97.
24. Ibid., p. 78.
25. Ibid., p. 77.
26. See L. Davidoff and C. Hall, *Family Fortunes: Men and Women of the English Middle Classes 1780–1850* (London: Routledge, 1992) for the most thorough history of family gender structure in the period that currently exists. See also A. Vickery, *The Gentleman's Daughter: Women's Lives in Georgian England* (New Haven, CT, and London: Yale University Press, 1998) for an account that argues that the lived familial relationships of people in the period were considerably more complex than the ideals set out in conduct literature and novels. Finally, see N. Armstrong, *Desire and Domestic Fiction: A Political*

History of the Novel (New York and Oxford: Oxford University Press, 1987) for an argument that situates conservative female subjectivities in the home as a primary cultural force in shaping the modern middle class.

27. Smith, *Ethelinde*, p. 68.
28. Ibid.
29. Ibid.
30. Ibid., p. 69.
31. Ibid., p. 290.
32. Ibid., p. 23.
33. Ibid., p. 290.
34. Ibid., p. 23.
35. Ibid., p. 290.
36. Ibid.
37. Ibid.
38. Ibid.
39. Ibid.
40. Ibid.
41. Ibid., p. 291.
42. Ibid., p. 50.
43. Ibid., p. 482.
44. Ibid., pp. 318–19.
45. Ibid., p. 319.
46. Ibid.
47. Ibid., p. 324.
48. Ibid., p. 319.
49. Ibid.
50. Ibid.
51. Ibid., p. 513.
52. Ibid., p. 329.
53. Ibid., p. 498.

2 McInnes, 'Amazonian Fashions: Lady Delacour's (Re)Dress in Maria Edgeworth's *Belinda*'

1. Thanks to the industrious editors of *Picturing Women's Health*, Fran Scott, Kate Scarth and Ji Won Chung, for their patience, enthusiasm and encouragement with this project.
2. M. Edgeworth, *Belinda*, ed. K. Kirkpatrick (1801; Oxford: Oxford University Press, 1999), p. 478.
3. See M. Butler, *Maria Edgeworth: A Literary Biography* (Oxford: Oxford University Press, 1972) for Butler's influential positioning of Edgeworth as a conservative writer, heavily influenced by the politics of her father, and C. Ó Gallchoir, *Maria Edgeworth: Women, Enlightenment, Nation* (Dublin: University College Dublin Press, 2005), for an analysis of Edgeworth's more complex relationship both to contemporary political movements in Ireland, Britain and the wider world, and her father's ideas.
4. M. Hallett, 'James Gillray and the Language of Graphic Satire', *James Gillray: The Art of Caricature*, ed. R. Godfrey (London: Tate Gallery Publishing, 2001), pp. 22–37, on pp. 35–6.

5. D. Donald, *The Age of Caricature: Satirical Prints in the Reign of George III* (New Haven, CT, and London: Yale University Press, 1996), p. 41.
6. S. Greenfield, '"Abroad and at Home": Sexual Ambiguity, Miscegenation and Colonial Boundaries in Edgeworth's *Belinda*', *PMLA*, 112:2 (1997), pp. 214–28, on p. 218.
7. R. Perry, 'Colonizing the Breast: Sexuality and Maternity in Eighteenth-Century England', *Journal of the History of Sexuality*, 2:2 (1991), pp. 204–34, on p. 232.
8. Greenfield, 'Abroad and at Home', p. 219.
9. A. McCann, 'Conjugal Love and the Enlightenment Subject: The Colonial Context of Non-Identity', *NOVEL: A Forum on Fiction*, 30:1 (1996), pp. 56–77.
10. K. Kirkpatrick, '"Gentlemen Have Horrors upon the Subject": West Indian Suitors in Edgeworth's *Belinda*', *Eighteenth-Century Fiction*, 5:4 (1993), pp. 331–48.
11. Ó Gallchoir, *Maria Edgeworth*, p. 38.
12. S. Egenolf, *The Art of Political Fiction in Hamilton, Edgeworth and Owenson* (Farnham: Ashgate, 2009), pp. 73–104.
13. Edgeworth, *Belinda*, p. 32.
14. Perry, 'Colonizing the Breast', p. 218.
15. Quoted ibid., p. 222.
16. Quoted ibid., p. 220.
17. M. Wollstonecraft, *A Vindication of the Rights of Woman*, ed. M. Brody (London: Penguin, 2004), p. 177.
18. Edgeworth, *Belinda*, p. 42.
19. Ibid.
20. Ibid., p. 43.
21. Edgeworth, *Belinda*, p. 43.
22. See L. Moore, *Dangerous Intimacies: Toward a Sapphic History of the Novel* (Durham, NC: Duke University Press, 1997), 90–107.
23. Edgeworth, *Belinda*, p. 35.
24. Ibid., pp. 35–6.
25. Ibid., pp. 57–8.
26. See, for example, T. Michals, '"Like a Spoiled Actress Off the Stage": Anti-Theatricality, Nature and the Novel', *Studies in Eighteenth-Century Culture*, 39 (2010), pp. 191–214, which reads *Belinda* alongside Samuel Richardson's *Pamela* and Frances Burney's *Evelina*, as all three try 'to strengthen the novel's claim to social and critical respectability by distancing themselves and their eponymous heroines from theatricality', p. 192.
27. T. F. Robinson, '"Life is a Tragicomedy!": Maria Edgeworth's Belinda and the Staging of the Realist Novel', *Nineteenth-Century Literature*, 67:2 (2012), pp. 139–76.
28. Edgeworth, *Belinda*, p. 58 (original emphasis).
29. Ibid., pp. 64–5.
30. Ibid., p. 65.
31. Ibid.
32. J. Wesley, 'Admonitions', in *Collected Works of John Wesley*, vol. 11 (London: Thomas Cordeux, 1812), pp. 368–70.
33. Edgeworth, *Belinda*, p. 270.
34. R. Polwhele, *Anecdotes of Methodism* (London: Cadell and Davies, 1800), pp. 65–7.
35. Polwhele's 'Ignorance with itching ears' is a biblical allusion to 2 Timothy 4, in which St Paul warns Timothy he will meet with people whose 'itching ears' deafen them to the truth of their doctrines because they prefer to follow dogma more aligned to their

own desires. This reference also works for the way Edgeworth represents the self-serving desperation of Lady Delacour's turn towards Methodism.

36. H. MacFadyen, 'Lady Delacour's Library: Maria Edgeworth's *Belinda* and Fashionable Reading', *Nineteenth-Century Literature*, 48:4 (1994), pp. 423–39.
37. See D. Weiss, 'The Extraordinary Ordinary Belinda: Maria Edgeworth's Female Philosopher', *Eighteenth-Century Fiction*, 19:4 (2007), pp. 441–61.
38. Edgeworth, *Belinda*, p. 209.
39. Ibid., p. 210.
40. Ibid., p. 472.
41. W. Godwin, *Memoirs*, in *Collected Novels and Memoirs of William Godwin*, ed. M. Philp, 8 vols (London: Pickering & Chatto, 1992), vol. 1, p. 122.
42. Edgeworth, *Belinda*, p. 388.
43. Ibid., p. 453.
44. Ibid.
45. Ibid., p. 369.
46. Ibid., p. 477.
47. Ibid., p. 478.
48. Egenolf, *The Art of Political Fiction*, p. 102.

3 Richardson, 'Transforming the Body Politic: Food Reform and Feminism in Nineteenth-Century Britain'

1. See, for example, J. Vernon, *Politics and the People: A Study in English Political Culture, c. 1815–67* (Cambridge: Cambridge University Press, 1993).
2. For discussions of the 'body politic' in England and France, see, for example, M. Gatens, *Imaginary Bodies: Ethics, Power and Corporeality* (London: Routledge, 1996) and A. de Baecque, *The Body Politic: Corporeal Metaphor in Revolutionary France, 1770–1800* (Stanford, CA: Stanford University Press, 1997).
3. K. Sharpe and S. Zwicker (eds), *Refiguring Revolutions: Aesthetics and Politics from the English Revolution to the Romantic Revolution* (Berkley and Los Angeles, CA: University of California Press, 1998), p. 16.
4. R. Porter, 'Medicine, Politics, and the Body in Late Georgian England', in Sharpe and Zwicker (eds), *Refiguring Revolutions*, pp. 217–40.
5. L. Rosner, *The Anatomy Murders: Being the True and Spectacular History of Edinburgh's Notorious Burke and Hare and of the Man of Science Who Abetted Them in the Commission of Their Most Heinous Crimes* (Philadelphia, PA: University of Pennsylvania Press, 2010).
6. O. Brownson, *An Address on Intemperance* (Keene, NH: J. and J. W. Prentiss, 1833), p. 32.
7. Hansard, House of Commons Debates, 3 August 1832, vol. 14, col. 1086.
8. J. Wallach Scott, '"A Woman who has Only Paradoxes to Offer": Olympe de Gouges Claims Rights for Women', in S. E. Melzer and L. W. Rabine (eds), *Rebel Daughters: Women and the French Revolution* (Oxford: Oxford University Press, 1992), pp. 102–20.
9. M. Fawcett, 'Broken Windows – and After', *Daily News*, 9 March 1912.
10. S. K. Kent, *Sex and Suffrage in Britain, 1860–1914* (Princeton, NJ: Princeton University Press, 1987).

11. This phrase comes from L. E. Nym Mayhall, *The Militant Suffrage Movement: Citizenship and Resistance in Britain, 1860–1930* (Oxford: Oxford University Press, 2003), p. 83. See also J. Vernon, *Hunger: A Modern History* (Cambridge, MA: Harvard University Press, 2007), ch. 3.
12. K. Gleadle, '"The Age of Physiological Reformers": Rethinking Gender and Domesticity in the Age of Reform', in A. Burns and J. Innes (eds), *Rethinking the Age of Reform: Britain 1780–1850* (Cambridge: Cambridge University Press, 2003), pp. 200–19.
13. For further discussion on the role of the household in female political culture, see S. Richardson, *The Political Worlds of Women: Gender and Politics in Nineteenth-Century Britain* (London: Routledge, 2013), esp. chs 1 and 2.
14. For more details on Anna Kingsford's life, see *ODNB* and A. Pert, *Red Cactus: The Life of Anna Kingsford* (Watsons Bay: Books and Writers Network, 2006).
15. *Lady's Own Paper*, 5 October 1872.
16. *Lady's Own Paper*, 12 October 1872.
17. A. Kingsford, *Health, Beauty, and the Toilet: Letters to Ladies from a Lady Doctor* (London: Frederick Warne and Co., 1886), pp. iii–iv.
18. N. Kingsford, *An Essay on the Admission of Women to the Parliamentary Franchise* (London: Trübner and Co., 1868), p. 4.
19. Ibid., pp. 5–6.
20. Ibid., p. 10.
21. A. Kingsford, 'Some Aspects of the Vegetarian Question', in A. Kingsford and E. Maitland (eds), *Addresses and Essays on Vegetarianism* (London: John M. Watkins, 1912), pp. 125–245, on p. 125.
22. A. Kingsford, 'Letters on Pure Diet', in Kingsford and Maitland (eds), *Addresses and Essays on Vegetarianism*, pp. 64–76, on pp. 64–5.
23. A. Kingsford, 'Addresses to Vegetarians', in Kingsford and Maitland (eds), *Addresses and Essays on Vegetarianism*, pp. 145–50, on pp. 145–6.
24. Kingsford, 'Some Aspects of the Vegetarian Question', p. 136.
25. A. Kingsford, 'A Lecture on Food', in Kingsford and Maitland (eds), *Addresses and Essays on Vegetarianism*, pp. 77–100, on p. 88.
26. Kingsford, 'Some Aspects of the Vegetarian Question', p. 137.
27. A. Kingsford, 'The Best Food for Man', in Kingsford and Maitland (eds), *Addresses and Essays on Vegetarianism*, pp. 101–12, on p. 111.
28. W. R. Greg, 'Why are Women Redundant?', *National Review*, 14 (1862), pp. 434–60 and F. Power Cobbe, 'What Shall We Do With Our Old Maids?', *Fraser's Magazine*, 66 (1862), pp. 594–610.
29. Gleadle, '"The Age of Physiological Reformers"', p. 209.
30. L. Leneman, 'The Awakened Instinct: Vegetarianism and the Women's Suffrage Movement in Britain', *Women's History Review*, 6 (1997), pp. 271–87.
31. Pert, *Red Cactus*, p. 46.
32. For more details on Annie Cobden-Sanderson's life see *ODNB* and S. Richardson, '"You Know your Father's Heart": The Cobden Sisterhood and the Legacy of Richard Cobden', in A. Howe and S. Morgan (eds), *Rethinking Nineteenth-Century Liberalism: Richard Cobden Bicentenary Essays* (Leicester: Ashgate, 2006), pp. 229–46.
33. E. S. Pankhurst, *The Suffragette Movement: An Intimate Account of Persons and Ideals* (London: [n.p.], 1931), p. 229.
34. *The Times*, 31 October 1906.

35. The letter was widely published including in the US. See, for example, 'Imprisonment of the English Woman Suffragists', *Public*, 9 (1906), p. 856.
36. M. Fawcett, *What I Remember* (London: T. F. Unwin, 1925), p. 187.
37. She outlined her experience in a letter to the editor of *The Times* following Mrs Pankhurst's similar treatment in 1912. *The Times*, 1 April 1912.
38. *The Times*, 2 January 1907.
39. *The Times*, 30 November 1906.
40. *The Times*, 28 May 1907.
41. *The Times*, 10 December 1906.
42. A. Cobden-Sanderson, *How I Became a Vegetarian* (London: Dove Press, 1908).
43. *The Times*, 6 July 1908.
44. F. Blizzard, 'The True Significance of Food Reform', *Herald of a Golden Age*, 10 (1905), p. 25.
45. 'Menus for School Children', *Review of Reviews*, 40 (1909), p. 178.
46. C. Shaw, 'Eliminating the Yahoo – Eugenics, Social Darwinism and Five Fabians', *History of Political Thought*, 8 (1987), pp. 521–44.
47. 'Menus for School Children', p. 178.
48. *The Times*, 7 December 1908.
49. M. McMillan and A. Cobden-Sanderson, *London's Children: How to Feed Them and How Not to Feed Them* (London: ILP Publications, 1909).
50. James Vernon has recently identified the scientific approach as critical in the delivery of school meals, terming the efforts to translate ethical considerations into administrative techniques, techno-politics. J. Vernon, 'The Ethics of Hunger and the Assembly of Society: The Techno-Politics of the School Meal in Modern Britain', *American Historical Review*, 110 (2005), pp. 693–725.
51. William Morris to Jane Morris, 16 January 1884, cited in *The Letters of William Morris to his Family and Friends*, ed. P. Henderson (London: Longman, Green and Co., 1950), p. 193.
52. *The Times*, 20 August, 28 August, 4 September and 13 September 1909.
53. *The Times*, 1 December 1913.
54. *The Times*, 4 November 1905.
55. *The Times*, 17 February 1909.
56. *The Times*, 20 April 1908.
57. F. M. L. Thompson, 'Cobden, Free Trade in Land, and the Road to the Abbey National', in Howe and Morgan (eds), *Rethinking Nineteenth-Century Liberalism*, pp. 68–79.
58. A. Cobden-Sanderson, *Richard Cobden and the Land of the People* (London: ILP Publications, 1909).
59. Ibid., p. 7.
60. *The Times*, 28 June 1909.
61. Typescript of interview between Annie Cobden-Sanderson and the *Daily Chronicle*, 1904. Cobden Papers, West Sussex Record Office, Add. MS 6041.
62. *Lady's Pictorial*, 3 March 1888.
63. M. Caird, *Beyond the Pale: An Appeal on Behalf of the Victims of Vivisection* (London: William Reeves, 1896), p. 67.

4 Lewis, 'Stagnation of Air and Mind: Picturing Trauma and Miasma in Charlotte Brontë's *Villette*'

1. T. J. Graham, *Modern Domestic Medicine* (London: Simpkin and Marshall et al., 1826). Patrick Brontë's copy of the 1826 edition is held at the Brontë Parsonage Museum, Haworth. By the tenth edition (1848), in recognition of the centrality of 'disorders of the mind and nerves' to his enterprise, Graham includes an extended appendix of observations on the topic, which expands relevant entries from the 1826 edition. As it is not certain whether Patrick or Charlotte would have been aware of this appendix, the 1826 and 1848 editions are noted as such in subsequent references.
2. J. M. Caldwell, *Literature and Medicine in Nineteenth-Century Britain: From Mary Shelley to George Eliot* (Cambridge: Cambridge University Press, 2004), p. 97. In contrast, Emily Brontë's novel, *Wuthering Heights*, and choices during illness exhibit her distrust of medical intervention.
3. C. Brontë, *Villette*, ed. H. M. Cooper (1853; London: Penguin, 2004).
4. Ibid., p. 205.
5. Ibid., pp. 441, 451, 225.
6. See particularly Caldwell, *Literature and Medicine* and S. Shuttleworth, *Charlotte Brontë and Victorian Psychology* (Cambridge: Cambridge University Press, 1996).
7. On trauma and memory in the work of Emily Brontë and the Brontës' scientific contemporaries, see further A. Lewis, 'Memory Possessed: Trauma and Pathologies of Remembrance in Emily Brontë's *Wuthering Heights*', in R. Barnett and S. Trowbridge (eds), *Acts of Memory: The Victorians and Beyond* (Cambridge: Cambridge Scholars Publishing, 2010), pp. 35–53. This research forms part of my wider project on the emergent discourse of mental trauma in nineteenth-century literature, culture and psychology.
8. J. Douglas, *On the Philosophy of the Mind* (Edinburgh: Adam and Charles Black; London: Longman, Orme, Brown, Green & Longmans, 1839), pp. 197, 202.
9. W. B. Carpenter, *Principles of Mental Physiology*, 2nd edn (1874; London: Henry S. King, 1875), p. 24. This was an expansion of the outline of psychology in the fourth and fifth editions of Carpenter's *Principles of Human Physiology* (1852 and 1855; first edition 1842). Although discussion of 'unconscious cerebration' first appeared in the fourth London edition of *Principles of Human Physiology* (London: John Churchill, 1853), p. 811, Thomas Laycock argued that he was the first to develop the concept in his earlier study of mesmerism and the 'reflex action of the cerebrum', published in the *Edinburgh Medical and Surgical Journal* in 1838.
10. V. L. Ryan, 'Fictions of Medical Minds: Victorian Novels and Medical Epistemology', *Literature and Medicine*, 25:2 (2006), pp. 277–97, on p. 283.
11. Brontë, *Villette*, p. 39.
12. 27 August 1850, *The Letters of Charlotte Brontë*, ed. M. Smith, 3 vols (Oxford: Clarendon Press, 1995–2004), vol. 2, p. 457.
13. The Brontë Parsonage Library holds a copy of the 1790 edition (London: J. F. & C. Rivington).
14. E. Young, *The Complaint: or, Night-Thoughts on Life, Death, & Immortality* (London: R. Dodsley, 1742; repr. Cambridge: Cambridge University Press, 1989, ed. S. Cornford), pp. 123–4.
15. A. Tennyson, *In Memoriam: Arthur H. Hallam*, ed. K. Hart (1850; 1907–8 edn, London: Folio Society, 1975), V.iii.11–12. As Hart notes, the work was rewritten and

arranged over almost seventeen years, and Tennyson continued to revise it until his death (p. 9).

16. Ibid., V.i.1–4.
17. Brontë, *Villette*, p. 55.
18. Ibid., p. 67.
19. Ibid.
20. Ibid., p. 57.
21. Ibid., p. 108.
22. Ibid., pp. 15, 274.
23. J. Gezari, *Charlotte Brontë and Defensive Conduct: The Author and the Body at Risk* (Philadelphia, PA: University of Pennsylvania Press, 1992), pp. 165–8.
24. J. É. Esquirol, *Mental Maladies: A Treatise on Insanity*, trans. E. K. Hunt (First publ. in French in 1838; Philadelphia, PA: Lea and Blanchard, 1845), p. 336; J. C. Prichard, *A Treatise on Insanity and Other Disorders Affecting the Mind* (London: Sherwood, Gilbert, and Piper, 1835).
25. Brontë, *Villette*, p. 196.
26. Ibid., p. 329.
27. Ibid., p. 196.
28. Douglas, *On the Philosophy of the Mind*, p. 196; T. Brown, *Lectures on the Philosophy of the Human Mind*, 4 vols (Edinburgh: W. and C. Tait; London: Longman, Hurst, Rees, Orme, and Brown, 1820). Brown's popular work on mental philosophy (by 1851 it had reached its nineteenth edition) is one of a number of such texts that would have been available to the Brontës at the Keighley Mechanics' Institute Library: see C. Whone, 'Where the Brontës Borrowed Books: The Keighley Mechanics' Institute Library Catalogue of 1841', *Brontë Society Transactions*, 11 (1951), pp. 344–58.
29. Brontë, *Villette*, p. 196.
30. J. Hughes, 'The Affective World of Charlotte Brontë's *Villette*', *SEL*, 4 (2000), pp. 711–26, on p. 716.
31. Brontë, *Villette*, p. 470.
32. Ibid.
33. Gezari, *Charlotte Brontë and Defensive Conduct*, p. 160.
34. Brontë, *Villette*, p. 341.
35. [Anon.], 'The Passions', *Journal of Psychological Medicine and Mental Pathology* (edited by F. Winslow), 3 (1850), pp. 141–64, on p. 163.
36. T. Laycock, *A Treatise on the Nervous Diseases of Women; Comprising an Inquiry into the Nature, Causes, and Treatment of Spinal and Hysterical Disorders* (London: Longman, Orme, Brown, Green, and Longmans, 1840).
37. J. G. Millingen, *The Passions; or, Mind and Matter: Illustrated by Considerations on Hereditary Insanity* (London: John and Daniel A. Darling, 1848), p. 160.
38. Brontë, *Villette*, p. 286.
39. Ibid., p. 205.
40. Ibid., p. 206.
41. Shuttleworth, *Charlotte Brontë and Victorian Psychology*, p. 239.
42. G. F. Drinka, *The Birth of Neurosis: Myth, Malady, and the Victorians* (New York: Simon and Schuster, 1984), p. 12.
43. J. Oppenheim, *'Shattered Nerves': Doctors, Patients, and Depression in Victorian England* (Oxford: Oxford University Press, 1991), p. 181.
44. Brontë, *Villette*, p. 276.

45. J. Conolly, *An Inquiry Concerning the Indications of Insanity* (London: John Taylor, 1830; repr. London: Dawsons, 1964), pp. 1–2.
46. Brontë, *Villette*, p. 276.
47. Ibid., p. 289.
48. Ibid., pp. 285, 288.
49. Ibid., p. 212.
50. Ibid.
51. H. Holland, *Medical Notes and Reflections*, 2nd edn, rev. (1839; London: Longman, Orme, Brown, Green, and Longmans, 1840), p. 603.
52. Brontë, *Villette*, p. 278.
53. Ibid.
54. Brontë, *Villette*, p. 42.
55. Ibid.
56. Brontë, *Villette*, pp. 48, 42.
57. Ibid., pp. 46, 48.
58. Ibid., pp. 42–3.
59. Ibid., pp. 42, 120.
60. Ibid., p. 121.
61. Ibid., p. 43.
62. R. Whytt, *Observations on the Nature, Causes and Cure of Those Disorders which have been Commonly Called Nervous, Hypochondriac or Hysteric, to which are Prefixed Some Remarks on the Sympathy of Nerves* (London and Edinburgh: Becket, De Hondt and Balfour, 1765), pp. 213–14.
63. Graham, *Modern Domestic Medicine* (1826), 3rd edn, much enlarged (London: Simpkin and Marshall et al., 1827), p. 214.
64. R. Burton, *The Anatomy of Melancholy*, 12th edn, 2 vols (London: Cuthell et al., 1821), vol. 2, p. 601. The Brontës' 1827 edition similarly observes that 'too much solitariness is cousin-german to idleness, and a principal cause of melancholy', p. 56.
65. 'This Lime-Tree Bower my Prison', in *The Complete Poetical Works of Samuel Taylor Coleridge*, ed. E. H. Coleridge, 2 vols (1797; Oxford: Clarendon Press, 1912), vol. 1, pp. 178–81.
66. Graham, *Modern Domestic Medicine* (1848), p. 16; see (1826), p. 394. Few are as quick as Graham wholeheartedly to recommend confinement (within asylum, or plain room) as expeditious 'cure' in the case of unsound mind.
67. Prichard, *A Treatise on Insanity*, pp. 288, 293.
68. Brontë, *Villette*, pp. 122, 119.
69. J. Reid, *Essays on Hypochondriasis, and Other Nervous Affections*, 3rd edn, rev. (1821; London: Longman, Hurst, Rees, Orme, and Brown, 1823), p. 81.
70. Ibid., p. 83.
71. Brontë, *Villette*, p. 532.
72. Reid, *Essays on Hypochondriasis*, p. 88.
73. Brontë, *Villette*, p. 173.
74. Reid, *Essays on Hypochondriasis*, p. 95.
75. Brontë, *Villette*, pp. 176, 174.
76. Ibid., p. 172.
77. Ibid., p. 173.
78. Reid, *Essays on Hypochondriasis*, p. 80.
79. Ibid., p. 88.

80. Brontë, *Villette*, pp. 39, 53.
81. Ibid., p. 296.
82. Ibid., p. 176.
83. Ibid.
84. Brontë, *Villette*, p. 50, 'cry': pp. 43, 176.
85. Holland, *Medical Notes*, pp. 499, 493.
86. G. M. Burrows, *Commentaries on the Causes, Forms, Symptoms, and Treatment, Moral and Medical, of Insanity* (London: Thomas and George Underwood, 1828; repr. New York: Arno Press, 1976), p. 471.
87. Brontë, *Villette*, p. 173.
88. Ibid., p. 176.
89. Caldwell, *Literature and Medicine*, p. 29.
90. H. Martineau, unsigned review, *Daily News*, 3 February 1853, p. 2, in E. McNees (ed.), *The Brontë Sisters: Critical Assessments*, 4 vols (Mountfield: Helm Information, 1996), vol. 3, pp. 589–90.
91. G. H. Lewes, '*Ruth* and *Villette*', *Westminster Review*, 59 (April 1853), pp. 245–54, in McNees (ed.), *The Brontë Sisters: Critical Assessments*, vol. 3, pp. 602–10, on p. 607.
92. Brontë, *Villette*, p. 542.
93. Ibid., pp. 545–6.
94. Ibid., p. 546.
95. Ibid., p. 39.
96. Ibid., p. 536.
97. Ibid., p. 176.

5 Wilson, 'The Iconography of Anorexia Nervosa in the Long Nineteenth Century'

1. 'Isabelle Caro dies after anorexia struggle', *Guardian*, 30 December 2010. In this essay, I use the adjective 'anorexic' to describe behaviour associated with the disease and the noun 'anorectic' to refer to a person suffering from anorexia nervosa. All italics used for emphasis and translations from French are my own unless otherwise indicated.
2. A search on Science Direct produced just 8 photographs out of 3,017 articles. None of the images appeared in high-profile journals such as the *Lancet*, the *British Medical Journal* [hereafter *BMJ*], or the *Annales médico-psychologiques*.
3. W. Gull, 'Anorexia Nervosa', *Transactions of the Clinical Society of London*, 7 (1874), pp. 22–8; C. Lasègue, 'De L'anorexie hystérique', *Archives générales de médecine*, 6 (1873), pp. 385–403.
4. J. J. Brumberg, *Fasting Girls: The History of Anorexia Nervosa* (New York: Vintage, 2000).
5. Brumberg offers three theoretical research models for anorexia: biological, psychological and cultural. The first is yet to offer 'a common biological characteristic of the anorexic population that is unambiguously a cause and not a consequence of extreme weight loss' (*Fasting Girls*, p. 28). The latter two are represented by Hilde Bruch and Susie Orbach, the two most influential thinkers on anorexia post-1960 – both psychoanalysts and pioneers in the search for meaning in the symptoms of anorexia.
6. Brumberg also discusses anorexia nervosa in the United States. The first picture of an anorectic was published in the US in the *New England Journal of Medicine* in 1936. This image, reproduced in Brumberg (*Fasting Girls*, p. 197), shows the patient from a

distance and is not a clinical photograph as such. Anorectics were not photographed in the same way as in England and France, however, and for this reason American cases are not discussed here.

7. Ibid., p. 213.
8. Freud links anorexia to 'a melancholia where sexuality is undeveloped' in an early paper from 1895. S. Freud, 'Extracts from the Fleiss Papers', in J. Strachey et al. (eds), *The Standard Edition of the Complete Psychological Works of Sigmund Freud, Vol. I (1886–1899): Pre-Psychoanalytic Works and Unpublished Drafts* (London: Vintage, 2001), pp. 175–282, on p. 200. Janet wrote about the problem of body image in his analysis of the case of Nadia, a young anorectic, in P. Janet, *Les obsessions et la psychasthénie* (Paris, 1903).
9. A. Morison, *The Physiognomy of Mental Diseases* (London: Longman and Co., 1840).
10. S. Gilman and H. Diamond, *The Face of Madness* (New York: Brunner/Mazel, 1976), p. 11.
11. M. First and A. Tasman (eds), *DSM-IV Mental Disorders: Diagnosis, Etiology and Treatment* (Chichester: Wiley, 2005), pp. 1101, 1110.
12. H. Bruch, *The Golden Cage: The Enigma of Anorexia Nervosa* (London: Harvard University Press, 2001). S. Orbach, *Hunger Strike: The Anorectic's Struggle as a Metaphor for our Age* (London: Karnac Books, 2005).
13. Orbach, *Hunger Strike*, p. xii. Although anorexia does affect men, fewer than 10 per cent of sufferers are male. The aetiology of the disease is considered to be different, and there are no examples of clinical photographs of anorexic men from the nineteenth century.
14. Examples of anorexia observed during wartime are reported in C. Poisson-Quinton, 'L'anorexie mentale: ses rapports avec la maladie de Simmonds' (Medical dissertation, University of Paris, 1943).
15. M. Lawrence, 'Anorexia Nervosa: The Control Paradox', *Women's Studies International Quarterly*, 2:1 (1979), pp. 93–101, on p. 100.
16. J. Ryle, 'Anorexia Nervosa', *Lancet*, 228 (1936), pp. 893–9, on p. 898.
17. S. Gilman, *Disease and Representation: Images of Illness from Madness to Aids* (Ithaca, NY: Cornell University Press, 1988), pp. 1–4.
18. For a detailed overview, see P. Wollen, 'On Gaze Theory', *New Left Review*, 44 (2007), pp. 91–106.
19. L. Mulvey, 'Visual Pleasure and Narrative Cinema', in L. Braudy and M. Cohen (eds), *Film Theory and Criticism* (Oxford: Oxford University Press, 2009), pp. 711–22, on p. 715.
20. Ibid., p. 718.
21. For Freud, 'scopophilia' is the 'normal' pleasure in looking that causes erotic arousal but which becomes a perversion (voyeurism) if it is 'connected with the overriding of disgust' or if 'instead of being *preparatory* to the normal sexual aim, it supplants it' (italics in original). See S. Freud, 'Three Essays on the Theory of Sexuality', in J. Strachey et al. (eds), *SE Vol. VII (1901–1905): A Case of Hysteria, Three Essays on Sexuality and Other Works* (London: Vintage, 2001), p. 157.
22. G. Flaubert, *Madame Bovary* (Paris: Michel Levy, 1857). C. Baudelaire, *Petits poèmes en prose* (Paris: Michel Levy, 1869).
23. Appetite is linked to the ideas of 'voice' and 'libido' in psychoanalytic writings, and is also described in these terms by Brumberg, who writes: 'The anorexic girl used both her appetite and her body as a substitute for rhetorical behaviour' (Brumberg, *Fasting Girls*, p. 165).

24. The images analysed in this section are taken from Gull, 'Anorexia Nervosa' (1874) and W. Gull, 'Anorexia Nervosa', in T. Dyke Acland (ed.), *A Collection of the Published Writings of William Withey Gull* (London: The New Sydenham Society, 1894), pp. 305–14.
25. Gull, 'Anorexia Nervosa' (1874), p. 24.
26. Ibid., p. 23.
27. G. Gasne, 'Un cas d'anorexie hystérique', *Nouvelle Iconographie de la Salpêtrière*, 13 (1900), pp. 51–6, on p. 51.
28. Gull, 'Anorexia Nervosa' (1874), p. 28.
29. Ibid., p. 22.
30. Ibid., pp. 25, 26.
31. T. Stretch Dowse, 'Anorexia Nervosa', *Medical Press and Circular*, 17 August 1881, pp. 95–7, 147–8, on p. 96.
32. Ibid., pp. 147, 148.
33. Ibid., p. 147.
34. Ibid., p. 148.
35. Ibid., p. 147.
36. W. Gull, 'Anorexia Nervosa', *Lancet*, 131 (1888), pp. 516–17, on p. 516.
37. Ibid., p. 517.
38. Brumberg, *Fasting Girls*, p. 121.
39. Bruch, *The Golden Cage*, p. 6. See also Orbach, *Hunger Strike*, p. xxii: 'anorexia exemplifies through the language of the body the woman's attempt to enter and at the same time disappear from a culture that derogates and deifies her'.
40. E. Brissaud and A. Souques, 'Délire de maigreur chez une hystérique', *Nouvelle Iconographie de la Salpêtrière*, 7 (1894), pp. 327–37. Brissaud was a professor of medicine based at the Saint-Antoine hospital, and Souques was a consultant in nervous illnesses at the Salpêtrière.
41. Ibid., p. 337.
42. Ibid., p. 329.
43. Ibid., p. 333.
44. Ibid., p. 334.
45. These journals contain many graphic images of deformed and disfigured patients with conditions such as elephantitis and acromegaly, as well as conjoined foetuses and extreme obesity.
46. S. Freud, 'The Uncanny', in J. Strachey et al. (eds), *SE Vol. XVII (1917–1919): An Infantile Neurosis and Other Works* (London: Vintage, 2001), pp. 217–56. 'Uncanny is what one calls everything that was meant to remain secret and hidden and has come into the open' (on p. 218).
47. H. Wallet, 'Deux cas d'anorexie hystérique', *Nouvelle Iconographie de la Salpêtrière*, 5 (1892), pp. 276–80.
48. Ibid., p. 276.
49. Ibid., p. 277.
50. Ibid., p. 278.
51. L. Stephens, 'Case of Anorexia Nervosa', *Lancet*, 145 (1895), pp. 31–2. First included as woodcuts in this paper, the original photographs are reproduced in Ryle's 1936 paper.
52. Ibid., p. 31.
53. Ibid., p. 32.

54. This painting is discussed in detail in the opening chapter of E. Bronfen, *Over her Dead Body: Death, Femininity and the Aesthetic* (Manchester: Manchester University Press, 1992).
55. Ibid., p. 5.
56. Black and white photograph of an emaciated woman, aged 17 years, suffering from 'hysteria', who refused food on account of anorexia (anorexia nervosa). Front view and back view, 1896, St Bartholomew's Hospital Archives and Museum, London, SBHU MU/14/49/16/1, 2, Wellcome Images.
57. Gasne, 'Un cas d'anorexie hystérique', p. 51.
58. Ibid., p. 53.
59. Wet nursing, involving long periods of separation from the infant's birth family, was common practice in all social classes in nineteenth-century France. For a more detailed discussion of wet nursing and its relevance to psychiatric case studies, see A. Hustvedt, *Medical Muses: Hysteria in Nineteenth-Century Paris* (London: Bloomsbury, 2011), pp. 225–6.
60. Gasne, 'Un cas d'anorexie hystérique', p. 52.
61. Evidence from England and Ireland shows that 'dry nursing' (i.e. artificial feeding) was normally fatal. An extreme example is that the Dublin Foundling Hospital was closed down because 99.6 per cent of 'dry-nursed' babies died. See V. A. Fildes, *Breasts, Bottles and Babies: A History of Infant Feeding* (Edinburgh: Edinburgh University Press, 1986), cited in G. Palmer, *The Politics of Breastfeeding* (London: Pandora, 1993), p. 185.
62. Gasne, 'Un cas d'anorexie hystérique', p. 53.
63. Ibid., p. 51.
64. Ibid., p. 53.
65. Some later photographs were found of patients suffering emaciation from organic causes. Significantly, however, despite reporting on anorexia the editors chose not to illustrate psychiatric illnesses. See H.-P. Klotz and J. Trémolières, *Les maigreurs: la dénutrition et l'anorexie mentale* (Paris: Expansion scientifique française, 1965).
66. G. Nogués, *L'anorexie mentale et ses rapports avec la psychophysiologie de la faim* (Toulouse: Dirion, 1913), p. 9.
67. These case studies are reported on pp. 149–58 (Miss M. C.) and pp. 159–62 (Miss G.) of Nogués, *L'anorexie mentale*.
68. Ibid., p. 158.
69. Ibid., p. 159.
70. Ibid., p. 160.
71. Ibid.

6 Sparks, 'Kate Marsden's Leper Project: On Sledge and Horseback with an Outcast Missionary Nurse'

1. Marsden also belonged to several respected associations, including the Royal British Nurses' Association (member and special badge holder) and the Russian Imperial Red Cross Society (member and medalist). K. Marsden, *On Sledge and Horseback to the Outcast Siberian Lepers* (New York: Cassell, 1892), frontispiece. Perhaps most prestigiously, she was among the first female fellows admitted to The Royal Geographical Society. E. Baigent, 'Kate Marsden', *Geographers Bibliographical Studies*, 27 (2008), pp. 52–69, on p. 63.

2. Marsden, *On Sledge and Horseback*, p. 3.
3. In the early 2000s journalist Felicity Aston travelled to the Sakha region in Siberia that Marsden documents, and was able to confirm the herb as kutchutka, a rare plant with unproven holistic efficacy. However, Aston discovered that an 1899 dictionary that translated the Sahka language to Russian states, after the entry for kutchutka, that 'This herb is used by the Yakut [Sakha] for curing leprosy'. F. Aston, 'Searching for a Miracle', *Geographical* (February 2008), at http://www.geographical.co.uk [accessed 5 November 2012], p. 38.
4. *ODNB*.
5. See, for instance, J. Swindells, *Victorian Writing and Working Women: The Other Side of Silence* (Cambridge: Polity Press, 1985); A. Easley, *First-Person Anonymous: Women Writers and Victorian Print Media, 1830–1870* (Farnham: Ashgate, 2004); A. Blunt, *Travel, Gender, and Imperialism: Mary Kingsley and West Africa* (New York: Guilford Press, 1994); M. Anderson, *Women and the Politics of Travel, 1870–1914* (Madison, NJ: Fairleigh Dickenson University Press, 2006).
6. C. Grogan exemplifies this approach even though her subject is eighteenth-century women writers: women 'often combined several genres within a single work [of fiction] to circumvent ... restrictive edicts about female intellect or propriety'. C. Grogan, 'Crossing Genre, Gender and Race in Elizabeth Hamilton's *Translation of the Letters of a Hindoo Rajah*', *Studies in the Novel*, 34 (2002), pp. 21–42, on p. 22.
7. Marsden, *On Sledge and Horseback*, p. 118.
8. Ibid., p. 185.
9. Ibid., p. 65.
10. R. Kipling, *Kim* (New York: Oxford University Press, 2008).
11. Marsden, *On Sledge and Horseback*, p. 11.
12. Ibid., p. 106. Other references to Marsden as a political infiltrator: pp. 11, 12, 126.
13. Ibid., p. 14.
14. Ibid., p. 24.
15. Ibid., p. 109.
16. Ibid., pp. 109, 56.
17. Ibid., p. 15.
18. Ibid., p. 38.
19. Ibid., p. 179.
20. Ibid., p. 195.
21. S. Mills, *Discourses of Difference: An Analysis of Women's Travel Writing and Colonialism* (New York: Routledge, 1991), p. 58.
22. Marsden, *On Sledge and Horseback*, p. 100.
23. Ibid., p. 36.
24. Ibid., pp. 35, 75.
25. Ibid., pp. 56–7.
26. Ibid., pp. 145, 146, 148. These grateful Siberians come from a wide range of social positions: they include a female domestic and two older men, one a leper and the other a doctor.
27. Marsden, *On Sledge and Horseback*, pp. 152, 215.
28. Ibid., p. 6.
29. Ibid., p. 69.

30. Ibid., p. 38. This statement describes Marsden's spearheading of the effort to clean the polluted river, not to help the lepers, but such language is consistent for all of the projects she takes on in the memoir, including her prison visiting and fundraising.
31. Ibid., p. x.
32. Ibid., p. 123.
33. Translation: a district police officer.
34. Marsden, *On Sledge and Horseback*, p. 141.
35. Anderson, *Women and the Politics of Travel*, p. 189.
36. Marsden, *On Sledge and Horseback*, p. 166.
37. Ibid., p. 162.
38. With its appendix and the report of her travels back to Moscow and St Petersburg, the text continues for another 124 pages.
39. Marsden, *On Sledge and Horseback*, p. 167.
40. Florence Nightingale insisted that nursing was a calling, not a career, and thereby helped to make it a more respectable 'outlet' (job) for middle-class women like Marsden. F. B. Smith, *Florence Nightingale: Reputation and Power* (London: Croom Helm, 1982). For lower-class nurses, like Dickens's slovenly Sairey Gamp in *Martin Chuzzlewit*, the profit motive and the degraded situations they were likely to occupy irreparably damaged nursing's 'womanly' associations.
41. Quoted in M. Vicinus, *Independent Women: Work and Community for Single Women 1850–1920* (Chicago, IL: University of Chicago Press, 1986), p. 117.
42. Marsden, *On Sledge and Horseback*, p. 69.
43. 2 John 4:35.
44. Marsden, *On Sledge and Horseback*, p. 268.
45. Ibid., p. 181.
46. Two historical examples from this era confirm the vulnerability of those who work on behalf of lepers. Father Damian (1840–89), the founder of the leper colony on Molokai, died from leprosy contacted there, and was beatified by the Catholic Church in 1995. (See J. Tayman, *The Colony: The Harrowing True Story of the Exiles of Molokai* (New York: Scribner, 2006)). Mary Reed (1858–1943), an American missionary, worked on behalf of the lepers in Chandag, India, where she contacted leprosy. (See G. H. Anderson, *Biographical Dictionary of Christian Missions* (Grand Rapids, MI: Wm. B. Eerdmans Publishing, 1999), p. 562.)
47. Marsden, *On Sledge and Horseback*, pp. 175, 212.
48. Ibid., pp. 116–17.
49. Ibid., p. 277.
50. Ibid., p. 159.
51. Ibid., p. 164.
52. Ibid.
53. Ibid., p. 226.
54. Other examples that I did not analyse here include Miss Mann and Miss Ainley in Charlotte Bronte's *Shirley*. Miss Mann becomes sick from her 'prolonged and unrelaxing attendance on the sick', and Miss Ainley 'would watch by any sickbed: she seemed to fear no disease'. C. Brontë, *Shirley* (New York: Penguin Classics, 1985), pp. 196, 197.
55. H. Martineau, *Deerbrook*, pp. 482–4.
56. Marsden, *On Sledge and Horseback*, p. 181.
57. E. Gaskell, *Ruth* (New York: Oxford University Press, 1985), p. 390.
58. Ibid., p. 425.

59. M. Poovey, *Uneven Developments: The Ideological Work of Gender in Mid-Victorian England* (Chicago, IL: University of Chicago Press, 1988), p. 165.
60. Marsden, *On Sledge and Horseback*, p. 197.
61. Ibid., p. 137.
62. Ibid., p. 117.
63. In the *ODNB*, Middleton cites the figure of £2,400.
64. F. Aston, 'Searching for a Miracle', p. 36.
65. Baigent, 'Kate Marsden', p. 69.
66. 'Help for Lepers', *BMJ*, 24 (December 1892), p. 1402.
67. Baigent, 'Kate Marsden', p. 70.
68. Ibid., p. 69.
69. Ibid., pp. 73–4.
70. Marsden, *On Sledge and Horseback*, p. 286.
71. Baigent, 'Kate Marsden', p. 71.
72. Ibid.

7 Ford, 'Constructs of Female Insanity at the *Fin de Siècle*: The Lawn Hospital, Lincoln, 1882–1902'

1. E. Showalter, *The Female Malady: Women, Madness and English Culture 1830–1980* (London: Virago, 1987; repr. 2008).
2. For example, see Victor A. Neufeldt's *ODNB* entry for Branwell Brontë, his published volumes of Branwell's writing, or Tom Winnifrith's work, including *The Poems of Patrick Branwell Brontë* (New York: New York University Press, 1983).
3. C. Alexander and M. Smith, 'Health of the Brontës', *The Oxford Companion to the Brontës* (Oxford University Press: 2006) Oxford Reference 2011, at http://www.oxfordreference.com/view/10.1093/acref/9780198662181.001.0001/acref-9780198662181-e-0516 [accessed 12 February 2013].
4. See Showalter, *The Female Malady*; L. Appignanesi, *Mad, Bad and Sad: A History of Women and the Mind Doctors from 1800 to the Present* (London: Virago, 2008; repr. 2009); or H. Small, *Love's Madness: Medicine, the Novel and Female Insanity 1800–1865* (Oxford: Clarendon Press, 1996).
5. M. Moore, 'Private vs. Public: Female Sexuality in Victorian Culture', at http://www.victorianweb.org/sculpture/nudes/1moore4.html [accessed 25 June 2013].
6. Appropriated from Coventry Patmore's 1854 (revised 1862) poem of the same title, on his wife, this term became shorthand for the ideal domesticated wife and mother, submissive to her husband.
7. Ibid., p. 26.
8. Ibid., p. 51.
9. M. S. Micale, *Hysterical Men: The Hidden History of Male Nervous Illness* (Cambridge, MA: Harvard University Press, 2008), pp. 5–6.
10. J. Oppenheim, *'Shattered Nerves': Doctors, Patients and Depression in Victorian England* (Oxford: Oxford University Press, 1991), p. 141.
11. The County Asylum at Bracebridge Heath opened in 1852 and catered for pauper and working-class patients.
12. The Lawn Hospital, Lincoln Interim Draft Catalogue, Lincolnshire Archives (Lincolnshire County Council, n.d.).

13. The Lawn Hospital presents an engaging case study because as a smaller asylum with a limited number of patients, it offered the potential for more direct interaction between doctors and those they treated. The archives therefore have a smaller scope for an overarching survey, but contain the potential for more detailed records of the individual patients admitted. Moreover, as the asylum primarily catered to upper- and middle-class individuals, and judging by nineteenth-century literary representations, this was the group most at risk of becoming the mad person or at least being mistaken for them, indicating some underlying truth in the cultural assumptions of society.
14. Appignanesi, *Mad, Bad and Sad*, p. 100.
15. Data taken from Lawn Hospital Admission Papers, 1882–1902, 1882 being the earliest date available.
16. 'Significant' meaning a difference of ten or more.
17. Admission Papers, 1882–1902.
18. Ibid.
19. C. F. Folsom, 'The Prevention of Insanity', *Public Health Papers and Records*, 7 (1881) pp. 83–90, at http://www.ncbi.nlm.nih.gov/pmc/articles/PMC2272425/ [accessed 13 July 2009], p. 86.
20. Admission Papers, 1882–1902.
21. For a literary take on this interpretation, also offering the direct voice of the patient, see Alexandra Lewis's 'Stagnation of Air and Mind' in this collection, pp. 59–76.
22. Lawn Hospital Visitor's Book, report dated 9 June 1885.
23. Data taken from Lawn Hospital Visitor's Book, October 1883.
24. Lawn Hospital Case Book 1880, p. 512.
25. Oppenheim, *'Shattered Nerves'*, p. 116.
26. M. Lawrence, 'Anorexia Nervosa: The Control Paradox', *Women's Studies International Quarterly*, 2:1 (1979), pp. 93–101.
27. S. Wilson, 'The Iconography of Anorexia Nervosa in the Long Nineteenth Century', this collection, pp. 77–104.
28. Lawn Hospital Case Book, 1880, p. 503.
29. Lewis, 'Stagnation of Air and Mind', p. 69.
30. Lawn Hospital Visitor's Book, Report dated October 1883.
31. Showalter, *The Female Malady*, p. 17.
32. Lawn Hospital Visitor's Book, Report dated June 1881.
33. Lawn Hospital Case Book 1900–1, page unknown.
34. Oppenheim, *'Shattered Nerves'*, p. 298.
35. H. Marland, *Dangerous Motherhood: Insanity and Childbirth in Victorian Britain* (Basingstoke: Palgrave Macmillan, 2004), p. 96.
36. Showalter, *The Female Malady*, p. 86.
37. Lawn Hospital Volume of Photographs, *c.* 1899, loose image.
38. Ibid.
39. Ibid., page unknown.
40. Lawn Hospital Case Book 1880, p. 503.
41. Lawn Hospital Volume of Photographs, *c.* 1899.
42. Ibid., page unknown.
43. Ibid., loose image.
44. Wilson, 'The Iconography of Anorexia Nervosa in the Long Nineteenth Century', p. 82.
45. Data taken from Registers of Removals, Discharges and Deaths 1873–90, 1890–5 and 1895–1906.

8 Brock, 'The Fitness of the Female Medical Student, 1895–1910'

1. Mrs I. Thorne, *Sketch of the Foundation and Development of the London School of Medicine for Women, Hunter Street, Brunswick Square, W.C.* (London: G. Sharrow, 1905), p. 43.
2. Ibid.
3. Ibid., pp. 44–5.
4. O. Wilberforce, *The Autobiography of a Pioneer Woman Doctor*, ed. P. Jalland (London: Cassell, 1989), p. 57.
5. Thorne, *Sketch*, p. 19.
6. Editorial, *BMJ*, 1:1799 (22 June 1895), p. 1394.
7. Editorial, *London (Royal Free Hospital) School of Medicine for Women Magazine*, 6 (January 1897), p. 213; 'RFH Magazine', *LRFHSMWM*, 42 (February 1909), p. 64. This publication will be abbreviated as *LRFHSMWM* in future notes. The periodical is extremely rare and the only full holdings are at the Royal Free Hospital Archives (afterwards RFHA), where the author consulted them.
8. Editors included Louisa Garrett Anderson (1897–1904) and Frances Ivens (1904–6). The Dean, Elizabeth Garrett Anderson, wrote in to the *Magazine* to ask for information to be submitted about medical practice among graduates working abroad. See *LRFHSMWM*, 20 (October 1901), pp. 839–40.
9. L. Kelly, '"Fascinating Scalpel-Wielders and Fair Dissectors": Women's Experience of Irish Medical Education, *c.* 1880s–1920s', *Medical History*, 54 (2010), pp. 495–516, on p. 498.
10. See K. Waddington, 'Mayhem and Medical Students: Image, Conduct and Control in the Victorian and Edwardian London Teaching Hospital', *Social History of Medicine*, 15:1 (2002), pp. 45–64; on p. 45.
11. 'Hospital and School News', *LRFHSMWM*, 23 (October 1902), p. 109.
12. For women's fight to enter the profession, see, for example, such classic accounts as E. M. Bell, *Storming the Citadel: The Rise of the Woman Doctor* (London: Constable, 1953) and M. A. Elston, 'Women Doctors in the British Health Service: A Sociological Study of their Careers and Opportunities' (PhD dissertation, University of Leeds, 1986).
13. Editorial, *Lancet*, 2:2605 (2 August 1873), p. 159.
14. From *North British Review*, 52 [1870], p. 333, in *Men-Midwives and Female Physicians; A Series of Extracts Showing the United Opinion of Many Eminent Medical Men, &c. On Both Subjects. Revised by a London Physician* (London: Job Caudwell, n.d. (post 1870)), pp. 34–5.
15. Letters, Notes &c: 'The Missing Lady Doctor', *BMJ*, 2:2231 (3 October 1903), p. 868. This case will be discussed at greater length in a forthcoming article of mine on 'The Death of Sophia Frances Hickman, M.D.' The stance of the popular press in this instance belies Anne Digby's comment that, generally, the 'non-medical press' were the ones expressing a 'sympathetic tone' towards medical women. See *The Evolution of British General Practice, 1850–1948* (Oxford: Oxford University Press, 1999), p. 156.
16. See 'The Death of Miss Hickman', *The Times*, 37219 (Friday, 23 October 1903), p. 8 and 'The Death of Miss Hickman: The Inquest', *The Times*, 37231 (Friday, 6 November 1903), p. 4.
17. Editorial, *LRFHSMWM*, 26 (October 1903), p. 217.
18. 'The Late Miss Hickman, M.D.', *BMJ*, 2:2238 (21 November 1903), p. 1356.

19. 'The Cost of a Medical Education', *BMJ*, 2:1810 (7 September 1895), pp. 574–7, on p. 577.
20. 'Hospital and School News', *LRFHSMWM*, 19 (May 1901), p. 804.
21. Wilberforce, *Autobiography*. Having received a scant amount of formal education, Wilberforce had even less experience than most; her failure to pass examinations, despite persistence and dedication, is excruciatingly told in her book.
22. C. R. Bell Keetley, *The Student's Guide to the Medical Profession* (London: Macmillan and Co., 1878), p. 44. Garrett Anderson's chapter is entitled 'A Special Chapter for Ladies Who Propose to Study Medicine' and can be found on pp. 42–8.
23. Ibid., p. 48.
24. Ibid., p. 9.
25. Ibid., p. 46.
26. For more on this transformation, see Waddington, 'Mayhem and Medical Students' and T. N. Bonner, *Becoming a Physician: Medical Education in Britain, France, Germany, and the United States, 1750–1945* (Baltimore, MD: The Johns Hopkins University Press, 2000), esp. chs 8 to 12.
27. 'The Cost of a Medical Education', p. 575.
28. For the vulnerability of the medical body, see, for example, R. Woods, 'Physician Heal Thyself: The Health and Mortality of Victorian Doctors', *Social History of Medicine*, 9:1 (1996), pp. 1–30 and C. Brock, 'The *Lancet* and the Campaign Against Women Doctors, 1860–1880', in A. M. Caleb (ed.), *(Re)Creating Science in Nineteenth-Century Britain* (Newcastle: Cambridge Scholars' Publishing, 2007), pp. 130–45.
29. See, for example, I. Zweiniger-Bargielowska, *Managing the Body: Beauty, Health and Fitness in Britain, 1880–1939* (Oxford: Oxford University Press, 2010).
30. 'The Cost of a Medical Education', p. 577.
31. A. Kenealy, 'How Women Doctors are Made', *Ludgate*, 4 (1897), pp. 29–35, on p. 32.
32. Waddington labels it a 'morally ambiguous zone', because of the social 'anxiety' surrounding death and dissection: see 'Mayhem and Medical Students', p. 53. See also C. Dyhouse, 'Driving Ambitions: Women in Pursuit of a Medical Education', *Women's History Review*, 7:3 (1998), pp. 321–43.
33. 'A Lover of Truth', 'Correspondence', *LRFHSMWM*, 23 (October 1902), p. 97.
34. Kenealy, 'How Women Doctors are Made', p. 33. For a different reading of how the Victorian middle-class nurse represented her self-sacrificing dedication to the profession, see Tabitha Sparks's chapter in this volume, 'Kate Marsden's Leper Project', pp. 105–18.
35. Figures compiled from *Register of Students* between 1895 and 1914, RFHA.
36. 'The London School of Medicine for Women', *Madame* (June 1898), pp. 782–4, *RFH Press Cuttings Book III*, RFHA. All quotations from pp. 783–4.
37. 'The London School of Medicine for Women. The Opening of the New Laboratories by the Princess of Wales', *London Argus: A Weekly Journal and Review of Municipal Life*, 3:61 (16 July 1898), pp. 162–3, on p. 163, *RFH Press Cuttings Book III*, RFHA.
38. Evidence of Mrs Elizabeth Garrett Anderson, M.D., 5 March 1891, *Select Committee of House of Lords on Metropolitan Hospitals, Provident and other Public Dispensaries, and Charitable Institutions for Sick Poor* (1890–1), 16452–531.
39. Statistics calculated from *Register of Students*, 1894–1911, RFHA, where departures are noted and sometimes reasons for bringing the course to an end. The eventual qualifications of each student are also marked, as is the date they qualify.

40. 'Notes, Short Comments and Answers to Correspondents', *Lancet*, 143:3680 (10 March 1894), p. 651. The *Daily News* also commented upon withdrawal statistics on 10 October 1907. See the *RFH Press Cuttings Book IV*.
41. Letter from 'M. B. L.' to Miss Brooks, 31 January 1913, in Student File: 'M. B. L.' RFHA.
42. Student Files for 'M. E. M'; 'C. B.'; 'F. K', RFHA. 'F .K.', however, features in the *LRFHSMWM* as having passed, in March 1912, the First Examination of the Royal College of Physicians, London, and Royal College of Surgeons, England. See 51 (July 1912), p. 83.
43. Special Meeting of the Council, 1 May 1901, *Minutes of the Council of the LRFHSMW*, SM 1/2/3/1, 1898–1912, RFHA.
44. Editorial, *LRFHSMWM*, 7 (May 1897), p. 270.
45. See Waddington, 'Mayhem and Medical Students'.
46. 'An Old Student' on 'Resignation of the Dean', *LRFHSMWM*, 25 (May 1903), pp. 163–4.
47. 'Some Notes on the Studentology of the Neighbourhood of Hunter Street and Gray's Inn Road (With Illustrations)', *LRFHSMWM*, 30 (January 1905), pp. 426–9.
48. 'The School Party, 1906', *LRFHSMWM*, 36 (February 1907), pp. 721–2.
49. The phrase is Kenealy's. For her account of an external visit, see 'How Women Doctors are Made', pp. 32–3.
50. 'Ward Entertainment', *LRFHSMWM*, 36 (February 1907), p. 730.
51. 'The Party', *LRFHSMWM*, 21 (January 1902), p. 903.
52. 'School News: The Summer Term', *LRFHSMWM*, 2 (October 1895), p. 77.
53. 'Hospital and School News: Annual Magazine Meeting', *LRFHSMWM*, 24 (January 1903), p. 149.
54. 'RFH Magazine', *LRFHSMWM*, 42 (February 1909), p. 65; 'The Magazine', *LRFHSMWM*, 27 (January 1904), p. 303.
55. 'RFH Magazine', *LRFHSMWM*, 42 (February 1909), p. 65.
56. 'Correspondence', *LRFHSMWM*, 22 (May 1902), p. 52. The first Annual Dinner was held at the end of 1902.
57. 'The Hospital Dinner', *LRFHSMWM*, 27 (January 1904), p. 300; 'The Annual Dinner', *LRFHSMWM*, 45 (February 1910), p. 215.
58. 'The Annual Dinner', *LRFHSMWM*, 30 (January 1905), p. 458.
59. In similar fashion to previous editors, Blair was already qualified: MB BS, BSc. She started editing the *Magazine* in October 1909 (issue 43). Blair's comments attracted the notice of the *Lancet*. See 'The Co-Education of Men and Women as Students of Medicine, 176:4532 (14 July 1910), pp. 112–13.
60. 'The Suggested Scheme of Opening the London Hospital to Women Students', *LRFHSMWM*, 46 (June 1910), pp. 267–8. Women were admitted to the London in 1918, but this was speedily revoked in 1921. See, for example, J. S. Gardener, 'The Great Experiment: The Admission of Women Students to St Mary's Hospital Medical School, 1916–1925', *Medical History*, 42 (1998), pp. 68–88.
61. E. W. Roughton, MD, FRCS, 'Opening Address at the London School of Medicine for Women: Women's Sphere in Medicine', *LRFHSMWM*, 47 (October 1910), pp. 292–305; esp. pp. 299–300.
62. 'Correspondence', ibid., pp. 326–7.
63. 'No, thanks very much', ibid., p. 238.

9 Marland, 'Unstable Adolescence/Unstable Literature? Managing British Girls' Health around 1900'

1. A. Kenealy, 'Woman as Athlete', *Nineteenth Century* (April 1899), pp. 635–45, on pp. 635, 641.
2. W. S. Playfair, 'The Nervous System in Relation to Gynaecology', in T. C. Allbutt and W. S. Playfair (eds), *A System of Gynaecology by Many Writers* (London: Macmillan and Co., 1896), pp. 220–31, on p. 221. Playfair was citing a leading article, 'The New Woman – Old Style', *Speaker* (12 January 1895), pp. 39–41, on p. 40.
3. *ODNB*.
4. E. E. Walker, *Beauty through Hygiene: Commonsense Ways to Health for Girls* (London: Hutchinson & Co., 1905), preface, p. 10.
5. Kenealy, 'Woman as Athlete', pp. 643, 645.
6. L. Ormiston Chant, 'Woman as an Athlete: A Reply to Dr Arabella Kenealy', *Nineteenth Century* (May 1899), pp. 915–19. For further details on this debate and the broader contestation of female athleticism, see H. Marland, *Health and Girlhood in Britain, 1874–1920* (Houndmills: Palgrave Macmillan, 2013), ch. 3; S. Fletcher, *Women First: The Female Tradition in English Physical Education 1800–1980* (London: Athlone, 1984); K. E. McCrone, *Sport and the Physical Emancipation of English Women 1870–1914* (London: Routledge, 1994).
7. [Anon.], 'What is the Chief End of Woman?', *Review of Reviews* (April 1899), p. 355.
8. In 1896 Playfair acquired a dubious reputation in an incident that shocked London society; he breached medical confidence when he revealed that his sister-in-law, Linda Kitson, had undergone an abortion while separated from her husband. Kitson sued Playfair for breach of professional confidence, and the public were riveted by the story of a middle-class woman's adultery being exposed by a man who was both her brother-in-law and physician. The resulting court case left Playfair £12,000 poorer, though unrepentant – Kitson was after all guilty of 'unchastity' – facing widespread public condemnation and a vitriolic press. In the long term it does not appear to have impacted on his career and financial well-being, *ODNB*. See, for Playfair, the essays by Hilary Marland and Chandak Sengoopta in M. Gijswijt-Hofstra and R. Porter (eds), *Cultures of Neurasthenia from Beard to the First World War* (Amsterdam and New York: Rodopi, 2001).
9. [Anon.], 'The Month', *Practitioner*, 55 (August 1895), p. 111.
10. Kenealy, 'Woman as Athlete', p. 643.
11. See K. Flint, *The Woman Reader 1837–1914* (Oxford: Clarendon, 1993).
12. A. Digby, 'Women's Biological Straitjacket', in S. Mendus and J. Rendall (eds), *Sexuality and Subordination: Interdisciplinary Studies of Gender in the Nineteenth Century* (London and New York: Routledge, 1989), pp. 192–220; see also, for example, C. E. Russett, *Sexual Science: The Victorian Construction of Womanhood* (Cambridge, MA: Harvard University Press, 1989).
13. W. S. Playfair, 'Note on the So-Called "Anorexia Nervosa"', *Lancet*, 1 (28 April 1888), pp. 817–8, on p. 818.
14. J. Mortimer-Granville, *Youth: Its Care and Culture. An Outline of Principles for Parents and Guardians* (London: David Bogue, 1880). See also D. Fowler, *Youth Culture in Modern Britain, c. 1920–c. 1970* (Houndmills: Palgrave Macmillan, 2008), pp. 18–19.
15. Mortimer-Granville, *Youth*, pp. 74, 79, 89–90, 95.
16. Ibid., p. 88.

17. G. Black, *The Young Wife's Advice Book; A Guide for Mothers on Health and Self-Management*, 6th edn (London: Ward, Lock and Co., 1888), p. 5.
18. E. J. Tilt, *On the Preservation of the Health of Women at the Critical Periods of Life* (London: John Churchill, 1851).
19. L. Weatherley, *The Young Wife's Own Book: A Manuel of Personal and Family Hygiene* (London: Griffith and Farran, 1882), p. 28.
20. Ibid., p. 30.
21. R. R. Rentoul, *The Dignity of Woman's Health and the Nemesis of its Neglect* (A Pamphlet for Women and Girls) (London: J. & A. Churchill, 1890), p. xxviii.
22. Ibid., pp. 45–6.
23. H. Marland, '"The Diffusion of Useful Information": Household Practice, Domestic Medical Guides and Medical Pluralism in Nineteenth-Century Britain', in R. Jütte (ed.), *Medical Pluralism: Past – Present – Future,* special issue of *Medizin, Gesellschaft und Geschichte*, 46 (2013), pp. 81–100; R. Porter (ed.), *The Popularisation of Medicine, 1650–1850* (London and New York: Routledge, 1992).
24. Flint, *The Woman Reader*, p. 53.
25. For girls' literature, see, for example, S. Mitchell, *The New Girl: Girls' Culture in England 1880–1915* (New York: Columbia University Press, 1995); M. J. Smith, *Empire in British Girls' Literature and Culture: Imperial Girls, 1880–1915* (Houndmills: Palgrave Macmillan, 2011); M. Beetham, *A Magazine of her Own? Domesticity and Desire in the Woman's Magazine, 1800–1914* (London and New York: Routledge, 1996); K. Drotner, *English Children and their Magazines, 1751–1945* (New Haven, CT, and London: Yale University Press, 1988).
26. See Marland, *Health and Girlhood*, ch. 2 for the diversification of this literature.
27. E. S. Chesser, *Physiology and Hygiene for Girls' Schools and Colleges* (London: G. Bell and Sons, 1914).
28. M. Morris (ed.), *The Book of Health* (London, Paris and New York: Cassell & Company, 1883).
29. H. Maudsley, 'Sex in Mind and in Education', *Fortnightly Review*, new series, 15 (April 1874), pp. 466–83.
30. E. Garrett Anderson, 'Sex in Mind and Education: A Reply', *Fortnightly Review*, new series, 15 (May 1874), pp. 582–94.
31. O. Moscucci, *The Science of Woman: Gynaecology and Gender in England 1800–1929* (Cambridge: Cambridge University Press, 1990), p. 104.
32. E. Clarke, *Sex in Education: Or, a Fair Chance for Girls* (Boston, MA: James R. Osgood, 1874), p. 18.
33. Ibid., p. 39.
34. Maudsley, 'Sex in Mind and in Education', pp. 468, 475–6.
35. H. Maudsley, *The Pathology of Mind: A Study of its Distempers, Deformities and Disorders*, 3rd edn of 2nd part of *The Physiology and Pathology of Mind* (London: Macmillan, 1879), p. 450.
36. The vast literature on hysteria includes S. Gilman, H. King, R. Porter, G. S. Rousseau and E. Showalter, *Hysteria beyond Freud* (Berkeley, CA: University of California Press, 1993); C. Smith-Rosenberg, 'The Hysterical Woman: Sex Roles and the Role Conflict in 19th-Century America', *Social Research*, 39 (1979), pp. 652–78; E. Showalter, *The Female Malady: Women, Madness and English Culture, 1830–1980* (London: Virago, 1987, 1st published New York: Pantheon, 1985), ch. 6; E. Showalter, *Hystories: Hysterical Epidemics and Modern Culture* (New York: Columbia University Press, 1997).

See also Flint, *The Woman Reader*, pp. 57–60 for the relationship between hysteria and reading, and for further examples of medical writing on the condition, P. Jalland and J. Hooper (eds), *Women from Birth to Death: The Female Life Cycle in Britain, 1830–1914* (Atlantic Highlands, NJ: Humanities Press International, 1986), section 2.4.

37. F. C. Skey, *Hysteria: Six Lectures Delivered to the Students of St. Bartholomew's Hospital, 1866* (London: Longmans, Green, Reader & Dyer, 1867), pp. 54–5.
38. Ibid., p. 55.
39. H. B. Donkin, 'Hysteria', in D. H. Tuke (ed.), *A Dictionary of Psychological Medicine* (London: J. & A. Churchill, 1892), pp. 618–27, on p. 620. See also S. Ledger and R. Luckhurst (eds), *The Fin de Siècle: A Reader in Cultural History, c. 1880–1900* (Oxford: Oxford University Press, 2000), p. 245.
40. Donkin, 'Hysteria', p. 620.
41. A. T. Schofield, 'Nervousness and Hysteria', *Leisure Hour* (June 1889), pp. 412–5, on p. 415.
42. A. Wilson, 'Plan Talks about Common Ailments and their Cures', *Health* (11 January 1895), pp. 226–7, on p. 226.
43. Tilt, *On the Preservation of the Health of Women*, p. 42; E. J. Tilt, *Elements of Health, and Principles of Female Hygiene* (London: Henry G. Bohn, 1852), pp. 141, 150–6.
44. J. H. Walsh, *Domestic Medicine and Surgery: With a Glossary of the Terms Used Therein* (London: Frederick Warne and Co, 1866), p. 167.
45. P. H. Chavasse, *Advice to a Mother: On the Management of her Children, and on the Treatment of the Moment of Some of their More Pressing Illnesses and Accidents*, 14th edn (London: J. & A. Churchill, 1889), p. 321.
46. Ibid., pp. 281–7.
47. W. S. Playfair, 'The Systematic Treatment of Functional Neurosis', in Tuke, *A Dictionary of Psychological Medicine*, vol. 2, pp. 850–7, on p. 854.
48. Playfair, 'The Nervous System in Relation to Gynaecology', pp. 220–1.
49. W. S. Playfair, 'Remarks on the Education and Training of Girls of the Easy Classes at and about the Period of Puberty', *BMJ*, 2 (7 December 1895), pp. 1408–10, quotes on pp. 1408, 1409.
50. C. Dukes, MD, FRCP, 'The Hygiene of Youth', in T. C. Allbutt and H. D. Rolleston (eds), *A System of Medicine, Vol. 1* (London and New York: Macmillan, 1905), pp. 161–81, on p. 179.
51. 'Medicus', 'The Weather and Health', *Girl's Own Paper* (*GOP*), 8:354 (9 October 1886), pp. 23–4, on p. 23.
52. 'Medicus', 'Health, Strength, and Beauty', *GOP*, 11:557 (30 August 1890), pp. 758–9, on p. 758.
53. 'Medicus' (Dr Gordon-Stables, R.N.), 'Physical Culture for Girls', 21:1037 (11 November 1899), pp. 86–7, on p. 86.
54. 'Medicus', 'Health, Strength, and Beauty', p. 758.
55. 'Medicus', 'Health all the Year Round', *GOP*, 6:259 (13 December 1884), pp. 166–7, on p. 166.
56. Drotner, *English Children and their Magazines*, pp. 152–3.
57. 'Medicus', 'Common-Sense Advice for Working Girls', *GOP*, 6:267 (7 February 1885), pp. 295–6.
58. 'Medicus', 'A Plain Talk with Sensible Girls', *GOP*, 17:860 (20 June 1896), p. 597.
59. G. Stables ('Medicus'), 'Health', *GOP*, 22:1128 (10 August 1901), pp. 716–7, on p. 716.

60. Gordon Stables ('Medicus'), 'Man-Games that Murder Beauty', *GOP*, 27:1376 (12 May 1906), pp. 502–3, on p. 503.
61. 'The New Woman – Old Style', p. 40.
62. F. H. Richards, *Hygiene for Girls: Individual and Community* (London: D. C. Health, 1913), p. 9.
63. E. S. Chesser, *From Girlhood to Womanhood* (London, New York, Toronto and Melbourne: Cassell, 1913), pp. 45–6.
64. *ODNB*; G. Jones, 'Women and Eugenics in Britain: The Case of Mary Scharlieb, Elizabeth Sloan Chesser, and Stella Browne', *Annals of Science*, 51 (1995), pp. 481–501, on pp. 486, 487.
65. Jones, 'Women and Eugenics in Britain', p. 489.
66. E. S. Chesser, *Youth: A Book for Two Generations* (London: Methuen, 1928), p. 33.
67. Chesser, *From Girlhood to Womanhood*, p. 46.
68. E. S. Chesser, 'The Girl's Wasted Years', *Quiver* (June 1911), pp. 746–8, on p. 746.
69. Ibid.
70. E. S. Chesser, *Woman, Marriage and Motherhood* (London, New York, Toronto and Melbourne: Cassell, 1913), p. 253.
71. Chesser, *Physiology and Hygiene*, p. 86.
72. See I. Zweiniger-Bargielowska, *Managing the Body: Beauty, Health and Fitness in Britain, 1880–1939* (Oxford: Oxford University Press, 2010); B. Søland, *Becoming Modern: Young Women and the Reconstruction of Womanhood in the 1920s* (Princeton, NJ, and Oxford: Princeton University Press, 2000).

INDEX

For Product Safety Concerns and Information please contact our EU
representative GPSR@taylorandfrancis.com
Taylor & Francis Verlag GmbH, Kaufingerstraße 24, 80331 München, Germany

www.ingramcontent.com/pod-product-compliance
Ingram Content Group UK Ltd.
Pitfield, Milton Keynes, MK11 3LW, UK
UKHW021303190926
475701UK00009B/633
9780367875954